Monographs on Endocrinology

Volume 19

Edited by

F. Gross, Heidelberg · M. M. Grumbach, San Francisco
A. Labhart, Zürich · M. B. Lipsett, Bethesda
T. Mann, Cambridge · L.T. Samuels (†), Salt Lake City
J. Zander, München

P. Mauvais-Jarvis
F. Kuttenn
I. Mowszowicz

Hirsutism

With 32 Figures and 10 Tables

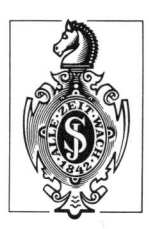

Springer-Verlag
Berlin Heidelberg New York 1981

Pierre Mauvais-Jarvis
Frédérique Kuttenn
Irène Mowszowicz

Department of Reproductive Endocrinology
Hôpital Necker
149, rue de Sèvres, 75730 Paris Cedex 15, France

Department of Biochemistry –
Faculty of Medicine Pitié-Salpétrière
75643 Paris Cedex 13, France

ISBN 3-540-10509-3 Springer-Verlag Berlin Heidelberg New York
ISBN 0-387-10509-3 Springer-Verlag New York Heidelberg Berlin

Library of Congress Cataloging in Publication Data.
Mauvais-Jarvis, P., 1929– . Hirsutism. (Monographs on endocrinology; v. 19)
Bibliography: p. Includes index. 1. Hypertrichosis. 2. Androgens –
Physiological effect. I. Kuttenn, F., 1944– joint author.
II. Mowszowicz, I., 1937– joint author. III. Title.
[DNLM: 1. Hirsutism. W1 MO57 v. 19/WR 455 M459 h]
RL431.M38 616.5'46 81–324
ISBN 0-387-10509-3 (U.S.) AACR1

This work is subject to copyright. All rights are reserved, whether the whole or part of the material is concerned, specifically those of translation, reprinting, re-use of illustrations, broadcasting, reproduction by photocopying machine or similar means, and storage in data banks. Under § 54 of the German Copyright Law where copies are made for other than private use, a fee is payable to 'Verwertungsgesellschaft Wort', Munich.

© Springer-Verlag Berlin, Heidelberg 1981
Printed in Germany

The use of registered names, trademarks, etc. in this publication does not imply, even in the absence of a specific statement, that such names are exempt from the relevant protective laws and regulations and therefore free for general use.

Typesetting, printing and binding: Oscar Brandstetter Druckerei KG, Wiesbaden

2125/3020– 543210

Preface

In the past 10 years hirsutism has been the object of a considerable number of fundamental studies. It provides endocrinologists with an experimental model for the investigation of androgen secretion, metabolism and mechanism of action. Plasma androgen assay, free testosterone measurement, hepatic and extrahepatic androgen metabolic clearance and androgen metabolism in the skin are the different steps which were studied by many groups and represent valuable parameters of the mechanisms of hirsutism.

Determination of the origin of androgen oversecretion has become easier by technical progress in differential effluent venous catheterism, which makes it possible to compare androgens in adrenal or ovarian effluent veins to their peripheral levels, and to determine the ovarian or adrenal source of the androgen oversecretion as well as the side responsible, essential in the case of tumors.

The study of androgen metabolism and the discovery of androgen receptors in the skin confirm the latter as an actual target cell for androgens. This target cell uses the circulating active androgen, i. e., testosterone and can also metabolize local inactive androgens into active ones. This is the case of androstenedione and dehydroepiandrosterone which are the two main androgens secreted in women, since women secrete very little testosterone. The capacity of the skin to transform inactive androgens into active ones varies from one individual to another. That would support the concept of variable skin receptivity from one woman to another and from one ethnic group to another. Skin receptivity is itself altered by circulating androgen levels. Androgen oversecretion and skin hypersensitivity are therefore closely interrelated pathologic phenomena.

Unfortunately, despite the considerable contributions of biochemistry to physiopathologic understanding of hirsutism, therapeutic means remain poor. It may be easy to suppress an androgen oversecretion in the case of a virilizing tumor, but it is more difficult to inhibit androgen oversecretion of nontumoral ovarian or adrenal origin which in any case will be incomplete. Moreover, skin "overuse" of circulating androgens often remains unaltered, even if the oversecretion is corrected. That is why the use of anti-androgens, active on the target cell itself, with good results, has now opened a new therapeutic era.

Pierre Mauvais-Jarvis
Frédérique Kuttenn
Irène Mowszowicz

Contents

A. Introduction 1

B. Androgen Control of the Pilosebaceous Gland 2

C. Androgen Production in Women 4
    I. Definition 4
    II. Androgen Biosynthetic Pathways 5
    III. Interconversion of Androgens 5
    IV. Plasma Levels and Blood Production Rates of Androgens 5
    V. Origin of Circulatory Androgens in Women 8
        1. Testosterone 8
        2. Androstenedione 8
        3. Dehydroisoandrosterone and Dehydroisoandrosterone Sulphate . 8
        4. Dihydrotestosterone 8
        5. Androstanediols 9
    VI. Control of Androgen Production in Women 9

D. Androgen Transport in Blood 11
    I. Testosterone-Binding Globulin 11
        1. Existence 11
        2. Purification of TeBG 11
        3. Characterization of TeBG in Serum 11
        4. Steroid-Binding Parameters of TeBG 12
    II. Other Plasma Proteins Binding Androgens 12
    III. Regulation of TeBG Activity 12
    IV. Physiological Role of TeBG Binding of Testosterone 13
        1. Relationship Between Testosterone Binding and Testosterone
           Metabolism 13
        2. Control of the Oestrogen-Androgen Balance in Women 13
        3. Selective Concentration of Active Molecules at the Target Cell Site 13

E. Hepatic Metabolism 15

F. Control of Plasma Level of Testosterone: Metabolic Clearance Rate . . . 16

G. Mechanism of Androgen Action in Human Skin 18

   I. Introduction 18
  II. 5α-Reduction of Testosterone into Dihydrotestosterone 19
      1. In Vivo Studies 19
      2. In Vitro Studies 20
         a) Biochemical Characterization 20
         b) Physiological Variations 20
         c) Control of Testosterone 5α-Reductase in Human Skin 20
         d) Pathological Models 23
         e) Studies with Cultured Skin Fibroblasts 24
 III. Dihydrotestosterone Formation from Other Androgen Precursors . 26
      1. Androstenedione 26
      2. Dehydroisoandrosterone 26
 IV. Intracellular Metabolism of Dihydrotestosterone 26
      1. Physiological Importance of 3α- and 3β-Androstanediols 26
      2. Characterization of the 3-Ketoreductases 27
  V. Intracellular Retention of Dihydrotestosterone 27
      1. Methodological Problems 27
         a) Cultured Fibroblasts 28
         b) Cell-Free Extracts 28
      2. Characterization of the Androgen Receptor 28
         a) Physiochemical Properties 28
         b) Heat Lability 29
         c) Dissociation Constant 29
         d) Specificity 29
      3. Physiological Variations 29
      4. Control of Androgen Receptor Concentration 30
      5. Pathological Variations 30
 VI. Conclusion 30

H. Clinical and Biological Assessment of Hirsutism 31

   I. Clinical Assessment 31
  II. Hormonal Investigation of Hirsutism 33
      1. Urinary 17-Ketosteroids 33
         a) Basal Conditions 33
         b) Tests of Ovarian Function 34
         c) Tests of Adrenal Function 34
      2. Plasma Androgens 35
         a) Assays of Testosterone 35
         b) Assays of Androstenedione 37
         c) Dynamic Tests for Plasma Testosterone and Androstenedione 37
         d) Ovarian and Adrenal Vein Catheterization 38
         e) Dihydrotestosterone 39
         f) Other Steroids 39

3. Evaluation of Androstanediols 40
4. Conclusion 41

I. Hirsutism of Adrenal Origin 43

I. Congenital Adrenal Hyperplasia Due to 21-Hydroxylase Deficiency 43
1. Introduction 43
2. Frequency 44
3. Pathophysiology 44
    a) General Remarks 44
    b) Single or Multiple Enzymes 45
4. Androgen Production in 21-Hydroxylase Deficiency 45
5. Clinical and Hormonal Characteristics of Delayed Onset Congenital Adrenal Hyperplasia Due to 21-Hydroxylase Deficiency 46
    a) Hormonal Data from the Literature 46
    b) Personal Data 47
    c) Interpretation of Results 50
6. Identification of the Heterozygous State 50
7. Genetic Linkage Between 21-Hydroxylase Deficiency and the HLA Blood Group System 51
8. Treatment 52
    a) Corticosteroid Replacement 52
    b) Other Treatments 52

II. Congenital Adrenal Hyperplasia Due to 11β-Hydroxylase Deficiency 53
1. Pathophysiology 53
2. Clinical Features 54
3. Hormonal Characteristics 54
4. Genetic Transmission 54
5. Treatment 54

III. Virilizing Adrenal Tumours 54
1. Pathology 55
    a) Macroscopy 55
    b) Histology 55
    c) Malignant Criteria 55
2. Steroid Production 55
    a) Dehydroisoandrosterone 56
    b) Other Androgens 56
3. Clinical Aspects of Virilizing Adrenal Tumours 56
    a) Adult Females 56
    b) Prepubertal Females 57
4. Hormonal Findings 57
    a) Urinary Steroids 57
    b) Plasma Steroids 57
    c) Dynamic Tests 57
5. Physical Methods for Diagnosis of Virilizing Adrenal Tumours . 58
6. Treatment 58

        a) Surgical 59
        b) Chemotherapy 59
        c) Benign Tumours 59

J. Hirsutism of Ovarian Origin 60

  I. Polycystic Ovarian Syndrome 60
    1. Theory of "Hypothalamic Masculinization" 60
    2. Two Types of Polycystic Ovaries 60
    3. LH-RH Test in the Polycystic Ovarian Syndrome 61
    4. Clomiphene Test 61
    5. Oestradiol Test 63
    6. Androgen Overproduction in Polycystic Ovarian Syndrome . . . 63
    7. Pathophysiology of Polycystic Ovarian Syndrome 64
    8. Treatment 66
    9. Conclusion 66
  II. Virilizing Ovarian Tumours 66
    1. Pathological Classification 67
        a) Arrhenoblastoma 67
        b) Hilus Cell Tumours 67
        c) Lipid Cell Tumours 67
        d) Granulosa and Theca Cell Tumours 68
        e) Gonadoblastomas 68
        f) Functional Stroma Tumours 68
        g) Luteoma 68
    2. Steroidogenesis 68
        a) Arrhenoblastoma 69
        b) Hilus Cell Tumours 69
        c) Luteoma 69
    3. Clinical Features 69
    4. Hormonal Investigations 70
        a) Assays in Basal Conditions 70
        b) Dynamic Tests 70
        c) Other Methods for Diagnosis 70
    5. Differential Diagnosis 71
    6. Prognosis 71
    7. Treatment 72
    8. Conclusion 72
  III. Ovarian Hyperthecosis 72

K. Idiopathic Hirsutism 74

  I. Basis of Androgen Hypersensitivity 74
  II. Hypersensitivity Versus Androgen Overproduction 75
  III. Clinical and Biological Characteristics 76
    1. Criteria for Estimation of Androgen Production 76

	2. Criteria for Estimation of Peripheral Androgen Consumption	77
	3. Personal Data	77
	a) In Vivo Studies	77
	b) In Vitro Studies	78
	c) Interpretation of Results	79
IV.	Treatment	81
V.	Conclusion	81

L. Treatment of Hirsutism 83

    I. Introduction 83

    II. Methods 83
        1. Oestrogens 83
            a) Mechanism of Action 83
            b) Clinical Use 83
        2. Progesterone 85
        3. Cyproterone Acetate 86
            a) Mechanism of Action 86
            b) Personal Results 86
        4. Corticosteroids 91

    III. Conclusion 91

References 92

Subject Index 109

Notations

Testosterone	: 17-β-Hydroxyandrost-4-en-3-one
Dihydrotestosterone	: 17β-hydroxy-5α-androstan-3-one
3α-Androstanediol	: 5α-Androstane-3α, 17β-diol
3β-Androstanediol	: 5α-Androstane-3β, 17β-diol
Androstenedione	: Androst-4-en-3, 17-dione
Dehydroisoandrosterone	: 3β-Hydroxy-androst-5-en-17-one
17-Hydroxyprogesterone	: 17-Hydroxypregnen-4-ene-3, 20-dione
HCG	: Human chorionic gonadotrophin
LH-RH	: LH, FSH releasing hormone
5α-Reductase	: Δ_4-3-Ketosteroid-oxidoreductase

A. Introduction

Hirsutism may be defined as an excessive growth of hair occurring in women on the face, chest, linea alba, buttocks and intergenitocrural regions, i.e. areas normally free of hair. Such hair growth may be present either without other abnormalities or be accompanied by other features of virilization such as hypertrophy of the clitoris, deepening of the voice, acne, breast atrophy, muscle hypertrophy, thinning of the scalp hair with temporal recession, and oligomenorrhoea or amenorrhoea. There is a direct relationship between the extent of hirsutism and the level of plasma testosterone in hirsute women (Table 1). Similarly, testosterone production rates increase in parallel with the severity of virilization, supporting the assumption that this potent androgen is largely responsible for virilization in women as in men. However, in most cases of hirsutism, plasma testosterone is either only slightly increased or within normal female range. Other biological parameters must also be considered in the pathogenesis of hirsutism: in particular, the role of the fraction of plasma testosterone which is not bound to specific proteins, the role of prehormones which may be transformed in the skin into active androgen, and the role of the target organ itself. There are clearly racial differences in the distribution of hair; facial hair is more common in Mediterranean women than in other European women, and very much more common than in Eastern women. No racial differences in parameters of androgenic steroids have been found, although they have been sought (Mansuwan and Kalant 1965).

Table 1. Correlation between plasma testosterone and clinical signs of virilization in hirsute women

Clinical findings	Plasma testosterone (ng/ml)
Normal women	$\leqslant 0.4$
Increased body hair	$\geqslant 0.6$
Facial hair	$\geqslant 0.8$
Menstrual disturbances	$\geqslant 0.9$
Clitoromegaly	$\geqslant 2.0$
Deepening of the voice	$\geqslant 2.5$
Increased muscle mass and/or balding	$\geqslant 3.5$

B. Androgen Control of the Pilosebaceous Gland

Numerous studies have established the dependence of sebaceous gland development on androgen. Sebum production levels in castrated men are considerably lower than in intact men (Strauss and Pochi 1963). However, the administration of testosterone to castrated males, children or postmenopausal women, in whom sebaceous secretion is normally low, results in a significant increase in sebaceous gland activity. The sebaceous gland is thus an androgen target organ (Pochi and Strauss 1974). Evidence that the sebaceous glands in women are less than maximally stimulated was suggested by studies in which the oral administration of methyltestosterone in daily doses of 100–200 mg sometimes produced a histologically detectable increase in sebaceous gland size (Strauss et al. 1962). In women with hirsutism, sebum excretion rate is higher when hirsutism is associated with acne, but there are many patients with extensive hirsutism in whom neither acne nor seborrhoea are observed. The problem regarding hair growth is more complex. The body surface of an infant, with the exception of the scalp and eyebrows, is covered with fine, soft, light-coloured hair; this is the vellus hair. Later in life, the hair at certain specific sites is replaced with longer, thicker and coloured terminal hair. This transformation of the vellus hair into the terminal hair appears to be governed by androgens. The amount of androgen necessary to effect this change depends upon a number of factors, Among them the race, sex and age of the individual and the site of the hair follicle on the body. Thus the transformation of pubic and axillary hair takes place under the influence of a small amount of androgen produced by normal women at the time of puberty. Larger amounts of androgen are required for the transformation of the hair follicles on the linea alba for example. Since all hair follicles of any one person are presumably subjected to the same androgenic stimulus, they must have different threshold levels of response. An intriguing problem remains to be solved: why are larger hairs produced by active androgens in some areas of the body whereas the hair follicles in the scalp in some individuals regress? Indeed, both sexual hair and male pattern baldness depend on androgenic hormones, in men as in women. In other words, why does testosterone (which on the face and some other regions of the body causes follicles to switch their hair production from vellus to terminal) have apparently the opposite effect in the scalp (Ebling 1976)? The response of sexual hair follicles to testosterone seems to be directly dependent upon its conversion to metabolites, of which dihydrotestosterone is the most important (Wilson and Walker 1969; Flamigni et al. 1971). By contrast, the action of dihydrotestosterone on the growth of scalp hairs may be differently mediated. Adachi et al. (1970) extracted adenyl cyclase from plucked growing scalp hairs; this is the enzyme responsible for producing cyclic AMP which is accepted as a common mediator of hormonal action at the cellular level and which is normally increased by hormonal stimulation. They showed that adenyl cyclase could be inhibited in vitro by dihydrotestosterone but not by testosterone, and they suggested that such a decrease would limit the energy metabolism and protein synthesis in scalp hair follicles in vivo. This hypothesis requires that bald skin converts testosterone to dihydrotestosterone more readily than hairy skin. The results of Bingham and Shaw (1973) support this possibility. These authors incubated male scalp skin from bald and hairy sites with ^{14}C-testosterone. In all four donors, both the uptake and the metabolism of testosterone were greater in the bald than in the hairy sites. Dihydrotestosterone formed about 20% of the total radioactivity.

All hair follicles undergo cycles of activity in which an active phase (anagen) alternates with a resting phase (telogen). The hair follicle cycle is controlled by both local and systemic factors. Each follicle has an intrinsic cycle characteristic of its region, but especially in respect to the initiation of anagen phase and, to a limited extent during activity, it is at the same time susceptible to hormonal systemic influences (Ebling 1976). In particular during the resting (telogen) phase, the initiation of anagen can be profoundly influenced by hormonal factors which can advance or retard it by several weeks. In humans, marked variations in the duration of anagen and telogen phases characterize different regions of the body (Saitoh et al. 1970); for example, for the scalp the duration of anagen and telogen phases averages 3 years and 3 months, respectively, and for the face 4 months and 2 months. It is thus essential that, in addition to considering linear growth rates of hair, such cycling be taken into account when attempting to interpret hair changes, or lack thereof, from hormonal or other manipulative treatments that could affect the hair follicle. There are, therefore presumably different threshold levels of response to androgens. There are also threshold variations with age, as with any biologically graded characteristic, and variations in sensitivity between normal individuals. These differences in end-organ sensitivity may have a basis in steroid biochemistry; they may particularly depend upon the rate of 5α-reductase enzymatic activity, permitting the conversion of testosterone to dihydrotestosterone and also upon the content in the philosebaceous gland of specific receptors binding dihydrotestosterone.

It is now technically possible to evaluate separately all the biological parameters involved in androgen action. In the light of results obtained, it may now be assumed that denomination of idiopathic hirsutism is inappropriate since most hirsutism, when correctly explored, is always accompanied by abnormalities suggestive of androgen secretion, blood production transport, and end-organ utilization.

C. Androgen Production in Women

I. Definition

Androgens have long been defined, on a physiological basis, as those molecules capable of stimulating the male reproductive tract. On a structural basis, all natural androgens are C 19-steroids with a flat junction between rings A and B and an oxygenated function on the 17th carbon (Fig. 1). Among these molecules, it is important to distinguish active androgens from inactive precursors or metabolites. Since knowledge of steroid mechanism of action has progressed, it has become possible to define active steroids on a molecular basis: only molecules capable of binding to the soluble intracellular androgen receptor with a high affinity can be considered active molecules; the others are either precursors or metabolites. Among the molecules presented in Fig. 1, only testosterone and dihydrotestosterone can be considered as active androgens. Androstenedione, which can be metabolized into testosterone both in the liver and target tissues, is an important precursor of active androgens.

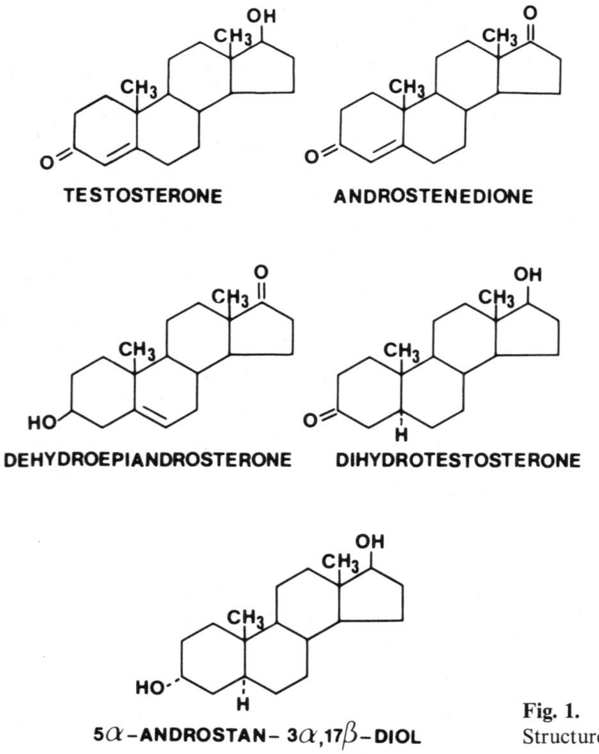

Fig. 1.
Structure of the main circulating androgens

II. Androgen Biosynthetic Pathways

A schematic representation of androgen biosynthetic pathways is given in Fig. 2. The human ovary contains all the enzyme systems necessary for testosterone synthesis (Ryan and Smith 1965). Even though androgens are important precursors of estrogens in the follicle, the studies by Rice and Savard (1966) have suggested that a major fraction of secreted ovarian androgens may be synthesized in the stroma. Further evidence of androgen secretion by the ovary is derived from the fact that their concentrations are five to ten times higher in ovarian vein plasma than in peripheral blood (Kirschner and Jacobs 1971; DeJong et al. 1974). The main androgens secreted by the adrenals are androstenedione and dehydroisoandrosterone (free and sulphate) (McDonald et al. 1965). However, some testosterone is directly secreted by the adrenals as shown by the gradient of concentrations between adrenal and peripheral veins (Kirschner and Jacobs 1971).

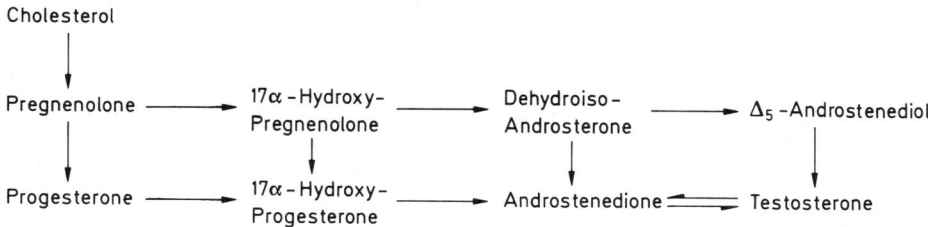

Fig. 2. Androgen biosynthetic pathways

III. Interconversion of Androgens

In addition to direct secretion, circulating androgens arise from peripheral conversion of secreted androgens. The interconversion rates between testosterone and androstenedione on the one hand, and dehydroisoandrosterone free and sulphate, on the other, have been calculated from studies involving administration of radioactive precursors (Horton and Tait 1966, 1967). These interconversions are especially important in women: they explain why blood production is higher than secretion rates (Figs. 3, 4).

IV. Plasma Levels and Blood Production Rates of Androgens

Testosterone, androstenedione, dehydroisoandrosterone and dehydroisoandrosterone sulphate are the major androgens produced and secreted into the circulation of normal women. Testosterone, the most active of these androgens, is five to ten times more potent than androstenedione and 20 times more potent that dehydroisoandrosterone (Dorfman and Shipley 1956) (Table 2).

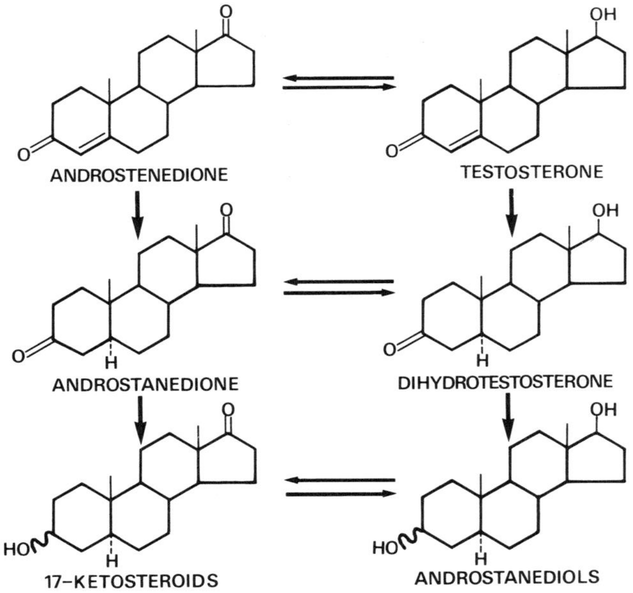

Fig. 3. Schematic metabolic pathways of active androgens

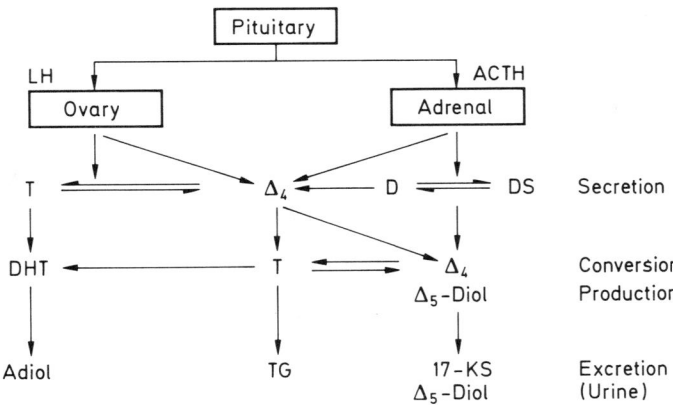

Fig. 4. General outline of androgen secretion, production and metabolism. T, testosterone; Δ_4, androstenedione; D, dehydroisoandrosterone; DS, dehydroisoandrosterone sulphate; DHT, dihydrotestosterone; Δ_5-Diol, 5-androstene-3β-17β-diol; 17-KS, 17-ketosteroids; $Adiol$, 3α-androstanediol; TG, testosterone glucuronide

Table 2. Normal values for major circulatory androgens in the blood of humans

	Testosterone			Androstenedione			Dihydrotestosterone			Androstanediol			
	Plasma C[a] (ng/ml)	MCR[b] (L/24 h)	PR[c] (mg/24 h)	Plasma C (ng/ml)	MCR (L/24 h)	PR (mg/24 h)	Plasma C (ng/ml)	MCR (L/24 h)	PR (μg/24 h)	Plasma C (ng/100 ml)	Urinary C[d] (μg/24 h)	MCR (L/24 h)	PR (mg/24 h)
Normal women	0.33 ±0.06	590 ± 44	0.23 ±0.07	1.40 ±0.21	2021 ± 110	3.0 ±0.5	0.18 ±0.03	200 ± 20	30 ± 10	2.6 ±0.5	44 ±24	1200 ± 200	35 ±10
Normal men	6.20 ±2.30	1240 ± 62	6.3 ±3.1	0.93 ±0.06	2027 ± 150	2.1 ±0.4	0.40 ±0.15	507 ± 50	150 ± 60	15.0 ± 5.0	200 ± 78	1600 ± 400	270 ± 50

[a] Plasma C, plasma concentration (mean ±SE).
[b] MCR, metabolic clearance rate (mean ± SE).
[c] PR, blood production rate (mean ± SE).
[d] Urinary C, urinary concentration (mean ± SE).

Table 3. Origin of plasma androgens in women

Steroids	Plasma concentration (ng/ml)	Secreted fraction		Fraction arising from peripheral conversion		
		Ovaries	Adrenals	From androstenedione	From testosterone	From DHEA
Testosterone	0.33 ± 0.08	10%–15%	10%–15%	50%–60%	–	16%–20%
Androstenedione	1.4 ± 0.2	60%	20%	–	< 1%	6%–10%
Dehydroepiandrosterone	3.2 ± 0.8	–	>80%	–	–	–
Dehydroepiandrosterone sulphate	0.9 ± 0.3	–	80%	–	–	20%
Dihydrotestosterone	0.23 ± 0.11		<1%	85%	15%	–

V. Origin of Circulatory Androgens in Women

Most of our knowledge of the origin of circulatory androgens is derived from various studies, including ovarian and adrenal vein catheterization (Kirschner and Jacobs 1971), and serum steroid levels throughout the menstrual cycle in normal women, with or without dexamethasone suppression (Abraham 1974; Vermeulen and Verdonck 1976), or after bilateral adrenalectomy (Abraham and Chakmakjian 1973) (Table 3).

1. Testosterone

Only 30%–40% of circulatory testosterone is secreted (Kirschner and Bardin 1972), half from the ovary and half from the adrenals. More than half of circulatory testosterone originates from peripheral conversion, the main precursor being androstenedione (Bardin and Lipsett 1967; Horton and Tait 1966; Vermeulen and Ando 1979). The major site of this conversion is not known; however, the liver is the location of 16%–30% of the androstenedione-to-testosterone conversion (Horton and Tait 1966; Rivarola et al. 1967a), and some of this metabolism can occur in blood (Blaquier et al. 1967). In addition, target cells for androgens, such as the skin (Wotiz et al. 1956) and skeletal muscle (Thomas and Dorfman 1964), possess the 17-ketosteroid reductase necessary to transform androstenedione into testosterone. This is of particular interest in the mechanism of action of androgens in these tissues; however, testosterone formed in these conditions is likely to be metabolized in situ and may never appear in the general circulation.

Peripheral conversion of dehydroisoandrosterone and 5-androstenediol to testosterone is not a significant source of testosterone in normal women (Kirschner et al. 1973).

2. Androstenedione

In contrast, around 80% of androstenedione arises from glandular secretion (Bardin and Lipsett 1967) and only 0.7% from peripheral conversion of testosterone (Horton and Tait 1966). The peripheral conversion of dehydroisoandrosterone to androstenedione accounts for only 6%–10% of circulatory androstenedione in normal women (Horton and Tait 1967; Kirschner et al. 1973). The ovaries secrete about two-thirds of androstenedione and the adrenals, about one-third (Abraham 1974).

3. Dehydroisoandrosterone and Dehydroisoandrosterone Sulphate

The adrenal supplies 80% of circulatory dehydroisoandrosterone and more than 80% of circulatory dehydroisoandrosterone sulphate (Abraham 1974).

4. Dihydrotestosterone

Dihydrotestosterone is the active androgen in most target cells. It is two to three times more potent than testosterone, although its production rate is only about one-fourth of that of testosterone, and it may represent an important factor of the androgen balance in women. It has been shown (Ito and Horton 1971; Mahoudeau et al. 1971) that this steroid is very rarely secreted by either the ovary or adrenals; thus plasma dihydrotestosterone mainly arises from peripheral conversion of prehormones. Androstenedione is the major precursor, testosterone contributing for only 15% of circulating dihydrotestosterone (Kirschner and Bardin 1972). Recent kinetic studies (Vermeulen and Ando 1969) have also shown that almost half of circulatory dihydrotestosterone could not be accounted for by peripheral conversion from androstenedione or testosterone, and these authors have suggested a possible role of dehydroisoandrosterone as an additional precursor.

In any event, plasma dihydrotestosterone probably does not reflect the presence of intracellular dihydrotestosterone, which is mainly formed in situ from testosterone 5α-reduction. As most androgen target cells contain 3-oxoreductases which actively metabolize dihydrotestosterone, cellular dihydrotestosterone is unlikely to be found in the plasma.

5. Androstanediols

3α- and 3β-androstanediols are the ultimate products of dihydrotestosterone reduction both in the liver (Tomkins 1956) and in target tissues, such as the prostate (Baulieu et al. 1968) or skin (Gomez and Hsia 1968; Wright and Giacomini 1980). It is still unclear whether they represent elimination products, or whether they can exert androgenic action either through back conversion to dihydrotestosterone or per se. The development of specific radioimmunoassays have allowed measurement of plasma androstanediols. Plasma concentrations of 3α-androstanediol are higher in men (range 120–180 pg/ml) than in women (range 25–30 pg/ml), and they are increased in hirsute women (Kinouchi and Horton 1974; Barberia et al. 1976; Laband et al. 1978; Meikle et al. 1979). Plasma concentrations of 3β-androstanediol are even higher (600–800 pg/ml in men, 300–400 pg/ml in women).
The sex difference is maintained and higher levels are also found in hirsute women (Hopkinson et al. 1977; Habrioux et al. 1978). Both steroids probably originate mainly from peripheral (hepatic and extrahepatic) conversion of dihydrotestosterone (Mahoudeau et al. 1971; Kinouchi and Horton 1974). Two remarks can be made concerning the origin of 3β-androstanediol. (1) Although the blood conversion rate of dihydrotestosterone to 3α-androstanediol is higher than the blood conversion rate of dihydrotestosterone to 3β-androstanediol (Mahoudeau et al. 1971), the higher levels of plasma 3β-androstanediol point to some other origin. (2) Hopkinson et al. (1977) measured the concentration of plasma 3β-androstanediol in two adult castrated males and as expected, this was reduced by two-thirds. However, no increase was observed after treatment with testosterone esters which restored normal plasma testosterone. As stated for dihydrotestosterone and as will be discussed further, the significance and physiological role of these androstanediols remain unknown and certainly requires more work.

VI. Control of Androgen Production in Women

The regulatory mechanisms that determine the production rate of androgens in women are ill defined. For the present, androgen secretion may be viewed as a by-product of oestrogen secretion by the ovary and corticoid secretion by the adrenal.

First, oestradiol and progesterone, and secondly cortisol, are the main glandular secretions involved in feedback of pituitary stimulins. The cyclic variations of testosterone and androstenedione concentrations during the menstrual cycle further support this view. Indeed, both steroids present higher values during the pre-ovulatory phase, which are not suppressed by dexamethasone (Judd and Yen 1973; Abraham 1974; Vermeulen and Verdonck 1976). By contrast, dehydroisoandrosterone free and sulphate are stable throughout the menstrual cycle (Abraham 1974). Thus, during adult life and in normal conditions, androgen secretion proceeds with, and in a way is controlled by, oestrogen and progesterone secretions. This is important as both oestradiol and progesterone have peripheral anti-androgen properties (see Sect. L.II.1, 2). However, there exist two periods in life, namely puberty and menopause, when this androgen/oestrogen balance is disrupted. At puberty, plasma levels of dehydroisoandrosterone start to rise in girls as young as 6–8 years old, whereas no increase in testosterone, oestrone or oestradiol is noted prior to 10–12 years of age and thereafter (Ducharme et al. 1976). The postmenopausal ovary secretes small amounts of oestradiol as shown by the measurement of ovarian vein levels of this steroid (Judd et al. 1974; Greenblatt et al. 1976). In contrast the ovarian stroma stimulated by high levels of gonadotropins continues to produce androstenedione and testosterone (Judd et al. 1974; Greenblatt et al. 1976; Maroulis and Abraham 1976). Surprisingly, plasma levels of dehydroisoandrosterone free and sulphate decrease drastically in menopausal women (Vermeulen and Verdonck 1978). These levels can be further suppressed by dexamethasone treatment (Maroulis and Abraham 1976). As no decrease in cortisol occurs at this period in life, it seems that regulatory mechanisms, other than ACTH stimulation, control the secretion of this steroid by the adrenals. At any rate, puberty as well as menopause, represents a period of relative hyperandrogenism, since target tissues are exposed to normal circulating levels of androgens, but unopposed by oestradiol and progesterone.

D. Androgen Transport in Blood

I. Testosterone-Binding Globulin

1. Existence

The existence of a plasma protein specifically binding testosterone was first suspected by Slaunwhite et al. (1959) and Chen et al. (1961) because of the higher binding affinity of testosterone to human serum, as compared to human albumin. Mercier-Bodard et al. (1965) first demonstrated that this protein was a globulin which bound testosterone with a high affinity. Subsequently, many investigators have confirmed the existence of this protein and have indicated that it binds other androgens and also oestrogens; thus, the name testosterone-oestradiol binding globulin (TeBG) was proposed (Pearlman and Crepy 1967; Vermeulen and Verdonck 1968; Mercier-Bodard and Baulieu 1968; Murphy 1968; Steeno et al. 1968; Corvol et al. 1971).

2. Purification of TeBG

The purification of TeBG has been difficult because of its very low concentration: around 2 mg per liter of plasma. Due to the development of affinity chromatography techniques it has recently been achieved (Renoir et al. 1977); this allowed the development of a radioimmunoassay for this protein (Mercier-Bodard et al. 1979). The measured concentrations are 4.02 ± 0.57 µg/ml in men, 8.21 ± 0.56 µg/ml in women.

3. Characterization of TeBG in Serum

In whole serum, gel filtration (Gueriguian and Pearlman 1968; Rosner et al. 1969) or gel electrophoretic studies (Corvol et al. 1971) indicated a molecular weight of about 100 000–115 000. No dissociation into active subunits could be produced by urea (Corvol et al. 1971). Isoelectric focussing experiments indicated the presence of considerable microheterogeneity (Van Baelen et al. 1969). It has recently been demonstrated (Vigersky et al. 1976) that the physicochemical properties of TeBG were very similar to those of the androgen binding protein (ABP) isolated from epididymal or sexual fluid in certain species. The significance of these similarities is still unclear, but it is of interest to note that the species distribution of these two proteins is quite different: in the human no evidence for ABP has yet been furnished, whereas in the rat for instance, there is ABP but no TeBG. The rabbit has both proteins (Mahoudeau and Corvol 1973; Danzo et al. 1974), but their physiological regulation is different, confirming the view that in spite of similarity, there are probably two different proteins.

4. Steroid-Binding Parameters of TeBG

The association constant of testosterone to TeBG decreases with temperature from 1.7×10^9 M^{-1} at 4° C (Mercier-Bodard and Baulieu, 1968) to $0.5–0.8 \times 10^9$ M^{-1} at 37° C (Vermeulen and Verdonck 1968; Dray 1969). The relative binding of other plasma androgens is as follows: dihydrotestosterone > 3α-androstanediol 3β-androstanediol > testosterone > oestradiol (Murphy 1968; Kato and Horton 1968). The presence of the 17β-hydroxy group is a necessary characteristic of steroids that bind to TeBG, and it must relate to a critical conformational structure of amino-acid residue at the binding site. It follows that steroids with a 17-keto group such as dehydroisoandrosterone, dehydroisoandrosterone sulphate and androstenedione do not bind to TeBG.

II. Other Plasma Proteins Binding Androgens

Transcortin, the specific binding protein for cortisol, corticosterone and progesterone also binds 17β-hydroxy androgens; however, at 37° C its affinity for androgens is very low and the amount of testosterone or dihydrotestosterone actually bound to transcortin in physiological conditions is negligible (Burton and Westphall 1972). The same applies to acid glycoprotein (Kerkay and Westphall 1968). In addition, albumin binds steroids with a low affinity (4×10^4 M^{-1} for testosterone) but with practically unlimited capacity. As a consequence, in normal women, about 75% of circulating testosterone is bound to TeBG, about 20% to albumin, and only 1% is free (Vermeulen et al. 1971).

III. Regulation of TeBG Activity

Variations in TeBG activity are observed in different physiological and pathological conditions. They affect the biosynthesis of the protein by the liver, as only the binding capacity is modified and the association constant remains the same (Dray 1969). Estrogens stimulate TeBG synthesis as shown by the higher levels found in women (binding capacity $8.02 \pm 2.67 \times 10^{-8}$ $M/1$) than in men ($5.51 \pm 1.76 \times 10^{-8}$ $M/1$) (Dray 1969). The level of TeBG increases two- to threefold during pregnancy (Pearlman et al. 1967) and after oestradiol treatment (De Moor et al. 1969; Vermeulen et al. 1969). In contrast, the lower TeBG binding capacity in men and hirsute women (Dray et al. 1968 a), and its higher level in androgen-insensitive patients with testicular feminization syndrome (Mauvais-Jarvis et al. 1970a) and hypogonadal men, (Dray 1969) indicate that androgens inhibit TeBG sythesis. Its level is also increased by thyroid hormone (Dray et al. 1967; Southren et al. 1969 b; Rosenfield 1971).

IV. Physiological Role of TeBG Binding of Testosterone

1. Relationship Between Testosterone Binding and Testosterone Metabolism

The following in vivo and in vitro studies support the contention that TeBG retards the metabolism of testosterone. In vivo it was noted that men who present lower TeBG levels than women have higher metabolic clearance rates (Bardin and Lipsett 1967; Southren et al. 1968). It was also noted that, in several clinical conditions such as virilism or hyperthyroidism, metabolic clearance rates are inversely correlated with changes in the binding capacity of TeBG (Vermeulen et al. 1969; Dray et al. 1968 b; Gordon et al. 1969). In contrast to testosterone, androstenedione is not bound to TeBG and is cleared from plasma twice as fast as testosterone. In species such as the dog and the donkey, which lack TeBG, testosterone and androstenedione are cleared from plasma at the same rate (Corvol and Bardin 1973). In vitro studies also confirm this assumption, e. g. binding of testosterone to TeBG inhibits aromatization by placental microsomes (Mowszowicz et al. 1970). It is of interest to note that high concentrations of albumin are equally effective in delaying testosterone aromatization by placental microsomes. This protein, in spite of its weak affinity, could also influence, through its high capacity, the transfer of testosterone to target or metabolic organs. Similarly, it has been shown that the presence of serum or purified plasma proteins in the culture medium influences the uptake and metabolism of testosterone by the prostate in constant flow organ culture (Lasnitski and Franklin 1975; Mercier-Bodard et al. 1976).

2. Control of the Oestrogen-Androgen Balance in Women

Another possible role for TeBG is the control of the oestrogen-androgen balance. Considering that both androgens and oestradiol bind to TeBG and have, moreover, opposite effects on this protein's synthesis, the following mechanism has been proposed by Burke and Anderson (1972): an increase in plasma testosterone could result in an increase of the free testosterone fraction, since androgens inhibit TeBG synthesis by the liver. However, testosterone which binds to TeBG with a higher affinity will displace oestradiol from its binding sites. The increase in free oestradiol in turn stimulates TeBG synthesis which is thus maintained. On the other hand, a rise in plasma oestradiol could tend to displace testosterone from its binding sites, thus increasing the free testosterone fraction. However, since there is a simultaneous increase in TeBG, the free testosterone fraction remains constant. This control is inadequate in women presenting at the same time an increase in testosterone and a decrease in oestradiol production, such as hirsute patients with anomalies of the menstrual cycle. In this case the relative or absolute hypoestrogenaemia may contribute to the development of hirsutism by potentiating the effect of testosterone (Tulchinsky and Chopra 1974).

3. Selective Concentration of Active Molecules at the Target Cell Site

This possibility was suggested by Robel (1971). The passage of testosterone across the cell membrane is a function of free testosterone concentration on each side of the membrane. In plasma, the only high affinity binder is TeBG. Within the target cell, testosterone is rapidly bound to a 5α-reductase and transformed into dihydrotestosterone, which in turn is bound either to the cytosolic receptor or to 3α- or 3β-ketoreductase and transformed into 3α- or 3β-androstanediols (see Sect. C.IV and V). These steroids will leave the cell and since they bind to TeBG with a higher affinity than testosterone, they can displace testosterone from its binding sites on TeBG. Free testosterone enters the cell, thus establishing a one-way circle where testosterone enters but never leaves the cell as such (Robel 1971).

E. Hepatic Metabolism

Like all steroid hormones, androgens are extensively metabolized in the liver. The metabolism results in inactive steroids which are thereafter eliminated mainly in the urine. Three types of reaction are essential: oxidation of the 17β-hydroxy group, reduction of the double bond and of the 3-keto group, and conjugation with glucuronic or sulphuric acid. Thus the main urinary metabolites of androgens are 17-ketosteroids with a reduced A ring. The existence of 5α-, 3α- and 3β-reductases has been demonstrated in the liver.

Although 17-ketosteroids are the major metabolites of testosterone, their excretion does not provide a reliable guide to the secretion of testosterone, since adrenal androgens are also metabolized and excreted largely as the same metabolites. Another better reflection of testosterone production is provided by the small proportion (1%) of testosterone which is excreted in urine, unchanged except for its conjugation with glucuronic acid.

Steroids formed in the liver are almost entirely conjugated with either sulphuric or glucuronic acid. As very little glucuronidase or sulphatase is present in the target tissues, it is very unlikely that steroids formed in the liver may ever have any biological action.

F. Control of Plasma Level of Testosterone: Metabolic Clearance Rate

As previously mentioned, there is no evidence to suggest that testosterone in women is maintained at a certain plasma level by an autoregulatory control, as it is in men via the pituitary Leydig cell axis. Therefore, the plasma concentration of testosterone can fluctuate not only with alteration of the production rate, but also with changes in the metabolic clearance rate. Since plasma testosterone may increase or decrease due to a change in clearance, it is obvious that the plasma level of this steroid is not always a good index of its production.

The control of the metabolic clearance rate of steroids is poorly understood. The role of protein binding and in particular binding to TeBG, has already been discussed. In view of the protective effect of this protein, one would assume that only the free steroid is available for metabolism. However, Baird et al. (1969) suggested that albumin-bound androgens were also metabolized, and they predicted that testosterone metabolic clearance rates would correlate with the quantity of free plus albumin-bound steroid. This was actually demonstrated by Vermeulen et al. (1969). However, this latter study also emphasized that factors other than plasma binding influenced the clearance rate of testosterone.

Testosterone metabolic clearance rates are greater in men (1200–1500 liters/24 h) than in women (600–800 liters/24 h) (Bardin and Lipsett 1967; Rivarola et al. 1966). Southren et al. (1968) demonstrated that the clearance rates in women could be increased to those found in men by chronic testosterone administration. In addition, Vermeulen et al. (1969) showed that the testosterone metabolic clearance rate in normal men was higher than in women, even when the amount of non-TeBG-bound testosterone was equal in the two sexes. These studies indicate that binding to plasma proteins is not the only factor regulating testosterone metabolism and that testosterone could increase its own tissue extraction. Another mechanism by which the rate of a steroid metabolism could be altered is the change in the activity of steroid-metabolizing enzymes. In the rat, testosterone and other drugs increase the activity of hepatic oxidative enzymes and the rate of steroid clearance from blood (Gillete 1967). A few drugs have been shown to increase hepatic enzyme activity in man. However, whereas medroxyprogesterone acetate treatment increases in parallel hepatic A-ring reductase and metabolic clearance rate (Gordon et al. 1970), N-phenyl barbital unexpectedly produced a small decrease in testosterone clearance in spite of the increased activity of several metabolizing enzymes (Southren et al. 1969a). Although the liver is recognized as a major organ for steroid biotransformation, there are many in vivo and in vitro studies suggesting important extrahepatic androgen metabolism. Thus the metabolic clearance rate can be viewed as the sum of hepatic and extrahepatic metabolism, which is mainly located in target organs for androgens. Hepatic metabolism of testosterone is not different in men or women; in contrast extrahepatic metabolism can be held responsible for the difference in metabolic clearance rate between the two sexes and thus plays an important role in the control of plasma testosterone, especially in women. It was first postulated (Bardin and Mahoudeau 1970) and then demonstrated (Kuttenn et al. 1977) that increased testosterone metabolism by extrahepatic target tissues, namely the skin, could explain the paradoxical occurrence of normal plasma testosterone levels in some virilized women with increased testosterone production rates.

G. Mechanism of Androgen Action in Human Skin

I. Introduction

The evidence of androgen action on human skin is multiple: the appearance of seborrhoea and hair growth at puberty, the excess of body hair in men as compared to women (in contrast to its absence in eunuchoid or hypogonadal men), and its development in women with adrenal or ovarian disease resulting in androgen hypersecretion. This hormone dependence affects mainly the philosebaceous gland (Strauss and Pochi 1963; Ebling 1976). However, the skin of the external genital organs also participates in their androgen dependency. Biochemically, human skin may be considered as a target organ for androgens, as are male accessory glands (see general reviews in: Mainwaring 1977; Liao 1977). Indeed, all events involved in testosterone action have been observed in this tissue (Fig. 5).

Thus, the 5α-reduction of testosterone into dihydrotestosterone, which seems to be an essential prerequisite for the action of testosterone in most target cells (Bruchovsky and Wilson 1968; Anderson and Liao 1968), takes place in the skin (Northcutt et al. 1969; Wilson and Walker 1969; Voigt et al. 1970). The presence of specific receptors for dihydrotestosterone in cultured human skin fibroblasts (Keenan et al. 1974) and in skin cytosol (Evain et al. 1977; Mowszowicz and Wright 1979) has also been reported. The intranuclear binding of dihydrotestosterone was observed in the sebaceous gland of the hamster (Takayasu and Adachi 1975) and in cultured human fibroblasts (Collier et al. 1978). In addition, the skin contains other enzymes capable of transforming inactive precursors into active androgens or of metabolizing dihydrotestosterone into 3α- or 3β-androstanediols. All these different proteins (enzymes and receptor) play an important role in regulating the in-

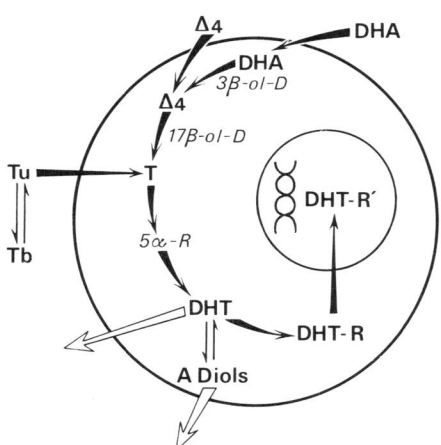

Fig. 5. Androgen metabolism and mechanism of action in human skin. *Tu*, testosterone; unbound testosterone; *Tb*, testosterone bound to TeBG; $Δ_4$, androstenedione; *DHA*, dehydroisoandrosterone; *3β-ol-D*, 3β-hydroxysteroid dehydrogenase; *17β-ol-D*, 17β-hydroxysteroid dehydrogenase; *5α-R*, 5α-reductase; *DHT*, dihydrotestosterone; *Adiols*, 3α- und 3β-androstanediols; *DHT-R*, DHT-cytosolic receptor complex; *R′*, nuclear receptor

tracellular concentration of dihydrotestosterone and hence the action of androgens in the skin. We shall now review the current knowledge on the activity and regulation of these different factors.

II. 5α-Reduction of Testosterone into Dihydrotestosterone

The 5α-reduction of testosterone is the most important step in the enzymatic processes involved in androgen action. The metabolism of testosterone in human skin was first demonstrated by Wotiz et al. (1956). After incubation of ^{14}C-testosterone with skin slices, these authors detected at least seven metabolites after chromatographic separation of the products, the main one being androstenedione. The most important study was carried out by Gomez and Hsia (1968), who found that the major metabolite of ^{14}C-testosterone was dihydrotestosterone; other identified metabolites were androstenedione, androstanedione, androsterone and isoandrosterone.

1. In Vivo Studies

Indirect information on testosterone metabolism by human skin was first obtained in the laboratory by in vivo experiments. The most interesting data were obtained by comparing the fate of radioactive testosterone simultaneously administered intravenously (^{14}C-testosterone) and percutaneously (^{3}H-testosterone) (Mauvais-Jarvis et al. 1969, 1970 a). The penetration of testosterone through the skin was established by dividing the ^{3}H : ^{14}C ratio of urinary 5β-androstanediol (which is presumably only formed by metabolism in the splanchnic compartment by the ^{3}H : ^{14}C ratio of radioactive testosterone, simultaneously administered by the percutaneous and intravenous routes. The absorption coefficient of ^{3}H-testosterone through the skin was around 10.0 ± 2.0 (SE) % of the administered dose (for 20 determinations). A coefficient, which enables the comparison of testosterone 5α-reduction by human skin from one subject to another, was calculated by dividing the ^{3}H : ^{14}C ratio of urinary androstanediol which originates from radioactive testosterone administration intravenously and percutaneously, by the ^{3}H : ^{14}C ratio of urinary 5β-androstanediol arising from the same precursors.[1] This coefficient may also be considered as the R value of androstanediol, taking into account the loss of ^{3}H-testosterone which results from its passage through the skin. In males, the corrected R value from androstanediol, i.e. the cutaneous coefficient for testosterone 5α-reduction, was around 2.4. In females it was less (very near to 1.0). It means that in this case the urinary yield of androstanediol is identical for testosterone administered either intravenously or percutaneously.

---

[1] Theoretical R value for androstanediol (Adiol) $= a \times \dfrac{1}{b}$ (in that case the absorption coefficient through the skin is assumed to be equal to 0.1).

$$a = \frac{^{3}H : {}^{14}C \text{ Adiol}}{^{3}H : {}^{14}C \text{ injection}}; \quad b = \frac{^{3}H : {}^{14}C \text{ 5β-Adiol}}{^{3}H : {}^{14}C \text{ injection}} = \text{absorption coefficient}$$

5β-Adiol (5β-androstanediol) is assumed to be exclusively of splanchnic origin.

2. In Vitro Studies

a) Biochemical Characterization

The 5α-reductase of human skin was further characterized by in vitro study (Voigt et al. 1970; Voigt and Hsia 1973). In contrast to what has been observed in the rat prostate, where about half of the enzyme activity was found in the nuclear membrane (Frederiksen and Wilson 1971; Moore and Wilson 1972), the maximum of 5α-reductase activity in human skin is localized in the microsomal fraction. The reaction is irreversible, requires NADPH as cofactor, and its optimal pH is 5.6. In contrast to the hepatic 5α-reductase which has a low specificity, the skin 5α-reductase seems much more specific. In addition to testosterone, it will reduce only deoxycorticosterone and, more importantly, progesterone which has an even higher affinity for the enzyme than testosterone itself. The dihydrotestosterone formed is further metabolized into 3α- and 3β-androstanediol.

b) Physiological Variations

Wilson and Walker (1969) were the first to study the regional variations in skin conversion of testosterone to dihydrotestosterone in detail. By incubation of ^{3}H-testosterone with slices of skin from various anatomical sites, they observed a wide variation in activity. The rate of dihydrotestosterone formation by the skin specimens from non-perineal sites (thigh, breast, back, leg etc.) was low (around 50 pmol/h/100 mg tissue), whereas in perineal tissue (prepuce, scrotum, labia majora, clitoris) dihydrotestosterone formation was considerably higher (50–1070 pmol/h/100 mg tissue).

Flamigni et al. (1971) have published additional results from the incubation of skin slices from healthy men and women with radioactive testosterone. These authors found a significantly higher conversion of testosterone to dihydrotestosterone and 3α-androstanediol in the scrotal skin of normal men (mean 37.2%), than in the abdominal skin (mean 4.7%). The difference in the recovery of dihydrotestosterone plus 3α-androstanediol from testosterone after incubation of the labia majora and abdominal skin of normal women was less important (7.8% and 5.9%, respectively). In addition, it has been demonstrated that dihydrotestosterone can be formed from testosterone in the skin of the face and back (Sansone and Reisner 1971), of the flexor and extensor aspects of the forearm (Rose et al. 1973), of the abdomen (Thomas and Oake 1974) and of the hair follicles themselves (Takayasu and Adachi 1972).

c) Control of Testosterone 5α-Reductase in Human Skin

α) *Pubic Skin*. In our laboratory, an extensive study was performed on 40 normal adult subjects, which concerned the suprapubic skin obtained during either laparotomy or biospy under local anaesthesia (Mauvais-Jarvis et al. 1974; Kuttenn and Mauvais-Jarvis 1975). Approximately 200 mg of each skin sample was incubated with ^{3}H-testosterone in the presence of an excess of NADPH. After homogenization, all skin specimens were incubated for 1 h at 37°C, and the calculation of metabolites recovered from radioactive testosterone included the sum of dihydrotestosterone plus 3α- and 3β-androstanediols. The mean recovery of 5α-reduced metabolites from testosterone incubated with skin from 20 normal men (Fig. 6) averaged 150 ± 30 fmol/mg, whereas in 20 normal women it was only 50 ± 10

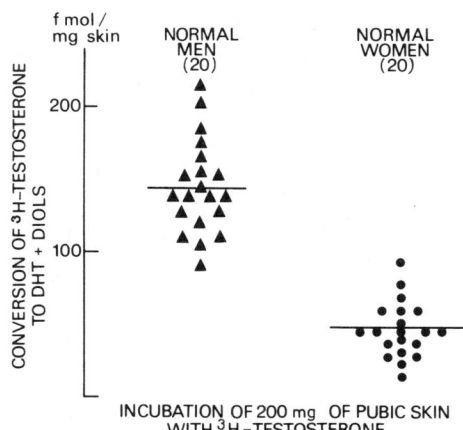

Fig. 6. Conversion to dihydrotestosterone (*DHT*) + androstanediols (*Diols*) of ³H-testosterone incubated with 200 mg pubic skin from normal adults. Kuttenn et al. 1980

fmol/mg skin. These two values are significantly different ($P < 0.001$). Such results differ from those obtained by Jenkins and Ash (1971), who found no male/female difference in the yield of dihydrotestosterone formed in pubic skin which had been incubated for 6 h with radioactive testosterone. However, the results of these investigators did not indicate the recovery of androstanediols from the skin homogenates. This would be interesting to know, since after 6 h of incubation of skin of normal men, the formation of androstanediols is higher than that of dihydrotestosterone (Fig. 7). We also think that the conflicting results obtained by different authors are caused mainly by the different experimental procedures used, in particular, the preparation of skin slices or homogenates, the supplementation with cofactors and the length of incubation.

The highest level of 5α-reductase activity measured in the pubic skin of men, as compared to women, could indicate a sex difference in the regulation of 5α-reductase activity in this area of the body, where it is well recognized that hair growth is under androgenic control.

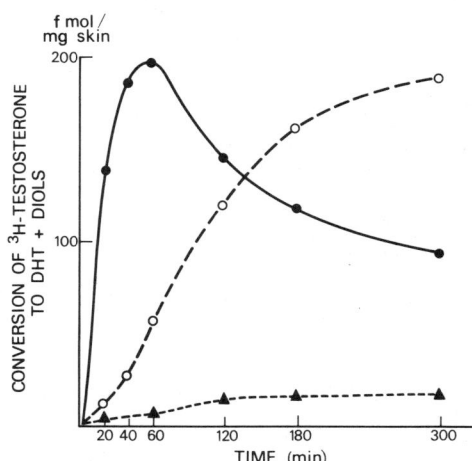

Fig. 7. Time course of formation of various metabolites of ³H-testosterone after incubation with 200 mg pubic skin from a normal man. *Solid line*, dihydrotestosterone; *dashed line*, androstanediols; *dotted line*, androstenedione; *DHT*, dihydrotestosterone; *Diols*, androstanediols. Kuttenn and Mauvais-Jarvis 1975

This would support the hypothesis that testosterone increases its own extrahepatic metabolism (Southren et al. 1968). To test this hypothesis, a systematic study (Kuttenn and Mauvais-Jarvis 1975) was conducted in hypogonadal patients and pre- and postpubertal children. The methods were as mentioned above for normal patients. Testosterone 5α-reductase activity in the skin obtained from children of either sex before puberty was very low (Fig. 8). In these subjects, the in vitro formation of dihydrotestosterone plus androstanediols by pubic skin ranged from 10 to 20 fmol/mg skin. These values are significantly lower than those of adult women ($P < 0.001$). In men, before the appearance of clinical symptoms of puberty (pubic hair growth and sebaceous gland activity), 5α-reductase activity increased dramatically. During the same period, plasma testosterone rose to about 3 ng/ml. In contrast, no change in 5α-reductase activity was observed in women during puberty.

A similar observation can be made in the case of hypogonadotropic hypogonadal males. 5α-Reductase activity is very low in the pubic skin of these patients, but increases dramatically after 3 weeks of treatment with human chorionic gonadotropin (hCG) at a daily dose of 1500 IU daily (Fig. 9). These results indicate that the 5α-reductase activity of pubic skin, involved in the appearance of secondary sex characteristics, is androgen dependent and can be an important step in the control of androgen action.

β) Genital Skin. Whereas 5α-reductase activity is higher in skin originating from external genitalia than in other areas, its control appears to be quite different. The enzymatic activity, as measured in vitro, is higher and similar in both sexes before puberty as well as after (Fig. 10) (Mauvais-Jarvis 1977). Siiteri and Wilson (1974) studied testosterone metabolism and dihydrotestosterone formation in the urogenital tract of differentiating human embryos. They found that 5α-reductase activity was present in the urogenital tubercle and urogenital sinus as early as the 1–3 cm stage, whereas it was undetectable in any other area of the skin (Flamigni et al. 1971). Thus, at the appearance of testosterone secretion by the fetal testis, dihydrotestosterone may be formed in the urogenital area and thus induces the male differentiation of these tissues. In the female fetus, 5α-reductase activity is present in external genitalia (clitoris, labia majora) (Wilson and Walker 1969; Flamigni et al. 1971), but in the absence of testosterone production, this activity remains quiescent

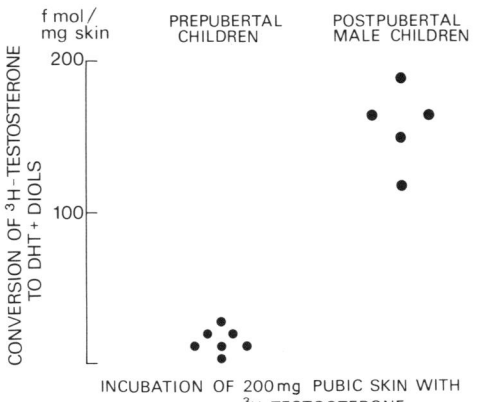

Fig. 8. Conversion to dihydrotestosterone (*DHT*) + androstanediols (*Diols*) of ³H-testosterone incubated with 200 mg pubic skin from prepuberal children and postpubertal males. Kuttenn et al. 1980

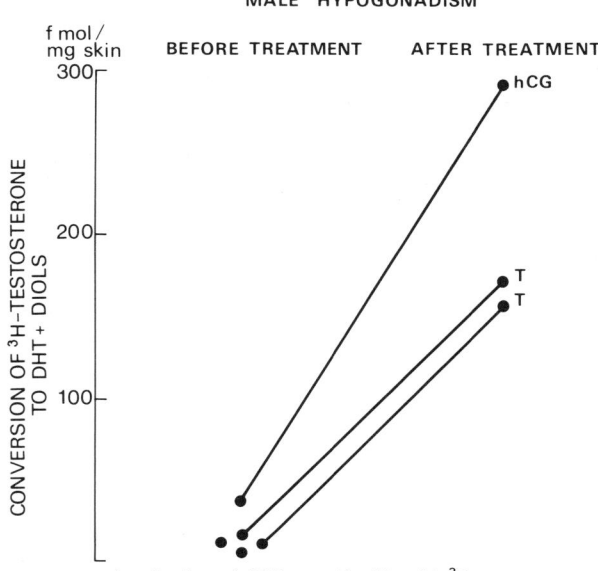

Fig. 9. Conversion to dihydrotestosterone (*DHT*) + androstanediols (*Diols*) of ³H-testosterone incubated with 200 mg pubic skin from hypogonadotropic hypogonadal men before and after treatment with HCG or testosterone (*T*). Kuttenn et al. 1980

for lack of substrate. Thus, in contrast to that observed in pubic skin, 5α-reductase in genital skin exists independently of androgen secretion and action.

d) Pathological Models

The importance of 5α-reductase during male sexual development and the dual type of control (for pubic and genital skin) is emphasized by the observation of patients

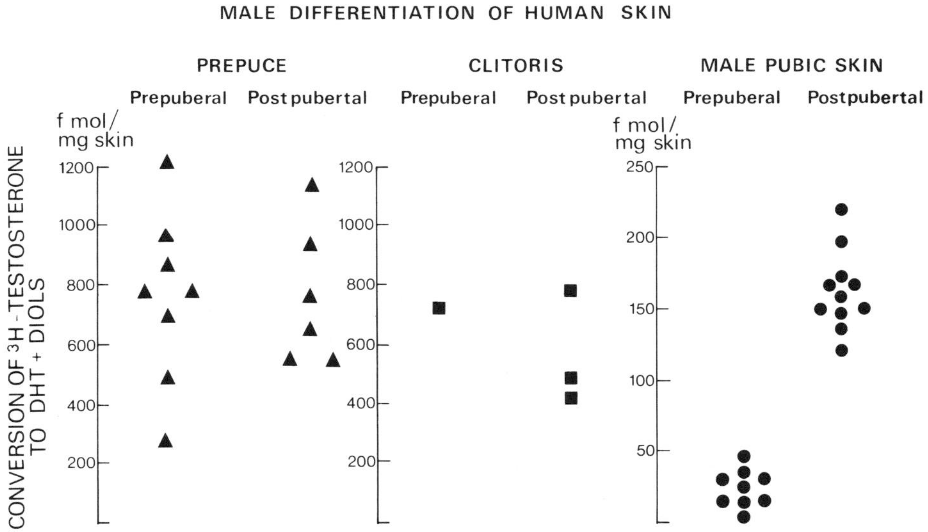

Fig. 10. Conversion to dihydrotestosterone (*DHT*) + androstanediols (*Diols*) of ³H-testosterone incubated with skin homogenates from various anatomical sites. Kuttenn et al. 1980

with abnormal sexual differentiation (Kuttenn et al. 1979b). Patients with the complete form of testicular feminization syndrome are completely insensitive to androgens due to the absence of the androgen receptor. These patients present a feminine phenotype and, at puberty, there is no appearance of body hair. The absence of 5α-reductase activity in the pubic skin of these patients is a consequence of their insensitivity to androgens, and is a further argument for the androgen dependence of this enzyme. In contrast, in perineal skin, 5α-reductase activity is normal, confirming that in this territory it is not dependent on androgen action. Male pseudohermaphroditism, due to 5α-reductase deficiency, was first described in 1974 by Imperato-Mc Ginley et al. It is characterized by the feminine differentiation of the external genitalia contrasting with the normal male differentiation of the wolffian derivatives. Patients with this syndrome have a normal androgen receptor concentration and no 5α-reductase in the perineal skin. That indicates that 5α-reductase is not androgen inducible in skin derived from urogenital tubercle and that it is an absolute necessity for the normal male differentiation of this territory.

e) Studies with Cultured Skin Fibroblasts

The 5α-reductase activity of human skin can also be studied in cultured skin fibroblasts. These cultures are easy to obtain and require very little cutaneous material. Tritiated testosterone can be directly incubated with fibroblast monolayers and the metabolites isolated from the medium. This technique is easy and presents the additional advantage of allowing one to explore functionally intact cells. Studies on 5α-reductase activity have been carried out in several laboratories (Shanies et al. 1972; Pinsky et al. 1974; Wilson 1975; Amrhein et al. 1977; Mowszowicz et al. 1980). In all these studies (in accordance with data obtained from incubation with skin slices or homogenates) the enzyme activity is higher in fibroblasts derived from foreskin, scrotum or labia majora than in pubic skin. Thus, cultured fibroblasts are functionally differentiated and represent valid models in the study of hormone metabolism and action.

Some results contrast with those of previous in vitro studies, in particular the large scattering of normal values (Leshin et al. 1978; Pinsky et al. 1978). In order to elucidate the reason for these discrepancies, we studied the 5α-reductase activity of cultured cell fibroblasts over a course of serial subcultures (Mowszowicz et al. 1980). When 5α-reductase activity was studied after the same number of subcultures for each strain, the results were in agreement with those obtained from skin homogenate incubations (Fig. 11) (Kuttenn and Mauvais-Jarvis 1975; Kuttenn et al. 1977). The fact that fibroblasts derived from different types of skin retain characteristic differences in 5α-reductase activity is further evidence that these differences are actually typical of the different types of skin. Thus, under certain conditions, 5α-reductase activity in skin fibroblasts reflects the physiological state of the skin they are derived from.

In the course of serial subculture, however, 5α-reductase activity increases, irrespective of the type of cell strain studied (Lamberigts et al. 1979; Mowszowicz et al. 1980). It is therefore clear that if cultures are studied after a variable number of subcultures, the results will be difficult to interpret. This point seems to us particularly important. Indeed, data in the literature always refer to assays performed between the "5th and 20th subculture". This may explain the wide range of values reported for cells from normal subjects and therefore the absence of

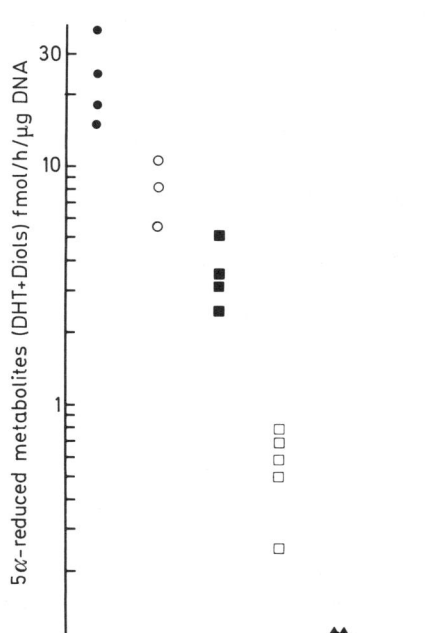

Fig. 11. 5α-Reductase activity of skin fibroblasts from normal foreskin (●) or pubic skin from normal men (○), normal women (□), hirsute women (■) and men with the complete form of testicular feminization syndrome (▲). Each point is the mean of triplicate incubations

significant correlations of 5α-reductase with various physiological and pathological conditions. In contrast, if cells are compared at the same age, the relative differences between the different skin types appear to be maintained.

The following hypotheses can be proposed to explain these variations in 5α-reductase activity:

1) Enzyme activity is *induced* by the steroids contained in the fetal calf serum. Preliminary data from our laboratory support this hypothesis: the addition of physiological concentrations of dihydrotestosterone to the medium of pubic-skin fibroblast cultures results in increased 5α-reductase activity; but in cells grown in the presence of charcoal-treated serum, 5α-reductase activity is reduced. However the increase of 5α-reductase in fibroblasts derived from foreskin (not androgen-dependent) and, moreover, from testicular feminization skin (a human model of androgen insensitivity) argues against this hypothesis.

2) A *modification* of the enzyme itself occurs, which alters its affinity for either the substrate or the cofactor. This would be in keeping with the reports of Leshin et al. (1978) who, in patients with pseudohermaphroditism due to 5α-reductase deficiency, found an enzyme activity within the low normal range in intact monolayers, but a decreased affinity for NADPH in cell homogenates. Cell cultures have also been shown to restore 5α-reductase activity in mouse kidney, whereas it is absent when measured in fresh tissue incubations (Mowszowicz and Bardin 1977).

3) *Selection* of an enzyme-rich cell population over the course of serial subculture occurs. There is indeed evidence for different metabolic pathways (Kaufman et al. 1975) or binding capacity (Meyer et al. 1975) in clones derived from the same cultures; it may therefore be that increased 5α-reductase activity represents an adaptive advantage for cells and that this selection is achieved through serial subculture.

In conclusion, whatever its cause, there is a regular increase in 5α-reductase activity of skin fibroblasts with serial subcultures. Due to the importance of this enzyme in physiological and pathological conditions, it is very important to point out that comparisons should be established only between cells of the same age (preferably early subcultures, as we do not know with certainty that the activity in all cells increases at the same rate). Taking this into account, cultured skin fibroblasts seem to retain the metabolic characteristics of the skin they are derived from and remain a very useful tool in the assessment of the androgen dependence of the skin.

III. Dihydrotestosterone Formation from Other Androgen Precursors

1. Androstenedione

Gomez and Hsia (1968) were the first to demonstrate that human skin is capable of converting androstenedione to testosterone and dihydrotestosterone. In a recent study by Flamigni et al. (1971) skin slices from genital and non-genital areas were incubated with radioactive androstenedione. Recovery of testosterone, dihydrotestosterone and 3α-androstanediol accounted for only 3%–4% of incubated androstenedione, whereas recovery of 5α-reduced metabolites of androstenedione (androstanedione and androsterone) was very high (around 50%). However, under in vivo conditions (Baulieu and Mauvais-Jarvis 1964), the proportion of androstenedione metabolized to dihydrotestosterone and androstanediols via testosterone is higher than during in vitro skin incubation with an excess of NADPH in addition to NAD.

2. Dehydroisoandrosterone

The conversion of dehydroisoandrosterone to testosterone by human skin was first demonstrated by Cameron et al. (1966) and additionally by Faredin et al. (1967), Gallegos and Berliner (1967) and Berliner et al. (1968). Recently, Thomas and Oake (1974) have reported that slices of skin from the linea alba of hirsute and normal women were able to convert radioactive dehydroisoandrosterone to testosterone, dihydrotestosterone and 3α-androstanediol. Thus, according to these investigators, human skin may be able, to transform dehydroisoandrosterone into testosterone and dihydrotestosterone, and variations in 3β-hydroxysteroid dehydrogenase activity may interfere with hair growth of sexual areas of the skin. The finding that skin is capable of forming testosterone (a potent androgen) from inactive androgens such as androstenedione and dehydroisoandrosterone is important. Skin thus appears to participate, not only in the catabolism of steroids, but also in the formation of active hormones from inert steroid precursors supplied through the blood (Mauvais-Jarvis et al. 1976a).

IV. Intracellular Metabolism of Dihydrotestosterone

1. Physiological Importance of 3α- and 3β-Androstanediols

Human skin has the ability to transform dihydrotestosterone into 5α-androstane-3α, 17β-diol (3α-androstanediol) and 5α-androstane-3α, 17β-diol (3β-androstanediol) (Wilson and Walker 1969; Gomez et al. 1972; Wright and Giacomini 1980). 3α- and 3β-ketoreductases are thus important enzymes which control the intracellular concentration of dihydrotestosterone in the androgen target cell. An increasing number of studies indicate that 3α- and 3β-diols might have androgenic actions per se: in the dog prostate, 3α-androstanediol is a better inducer of DNA polymerase than dihydrotestosterone (Harper et al. 1970), and 3α-androstanediol is six to eight times more effective than dihydrotestosterone in maintaining epididymal spermatozoid mobility in the castrated hamster (Lubicz-Nawrocki 1973). Moreover, the effect on LH secretion of 3α-androstanediol implants in the hypothalamus of castrated male rats is more important than that of dihydrotestosterone (Juneja et al. 1977). Despite the fact that the transformation of dihydrotestosterone to 3α-androstanediol is reversible in these tissues (Bruchovsky 1971), the stronger effects of 3α-androstanediol as compared to dihydrotestosterone indicate that back conversion to this latter steroid is probably not the sole mechanism of 3α-androstanediol action. In addition, in contrast to other androgen target tissues, 3α-keto reduction is not reversible in human skin (Wright and Giacomini 1980), and any effect of 3α-androstanediol should be a proper effect of this steroid.

The effects of 3β-androstanediol are even more convincing as it is generally recognized that 3β-keto reduction is irreversible in all androgen target tissues (Bruchovsky 1971; Mowszowicz and Bardin 1974; Wright and Giacomini 1980). In rat and human prostate, 3β-androstanediol stimulates cellular hypertrophy (Robel et al. 1971; Morfin et al. 1978); in castrated rats it stimulates sebaceous gland mitosis and secretion (Ebling et al. 1973) and modifies the composition of sebum (Nikkari and Valavaara 1970). It is the most important metabolite of testosterone in the scalp and back skin (Stewart et al. 1977) as these areas are particularly rich in sebaceous glands. It is not unlikely that modifications of 3β-androstanediol production might be responsible for increased sebum production in humans also.

2. Characterization of the 3-Ketoreductases

Recent in vitro studies (Wright and Giacomini 1980) have shown that 3α- and 3β-ketoreductases are present both in cytosolic and microsomal fractions of human skin; cofactors are NADPH and/or NADH, but 3α-ketoreductase has a higher affinity for NADPH whereas 3β-ketoreductase has a higher affinity for NADH. Factors regulating these two enzyme activities remain unknown.

V. Intracellular Retention of Dihydrotestosterone

1. Methodological Problems

Most of the dihydrotestosterone formed in target cells is bound to a soluble cytoplasmic protein named the "receptor". The steroid receptor complex is translocated into the nucleus and exerts its effects via an interaction with chromatin, leading to increased formation of mRNA (Mainwaring 1977; Liao 1977). The study of the androgen receptor in human tissues has been hindered by several specific problems: this protein has a somewhat lower affinity for its ligand than other steroid receptors, and it is extremely heat labile. But the main difficulty arises from the presence of plasma TeBG contaminating tissue samples, as the difference in affinities of the two proteins towards dihydrotestosterone is only three- to fivefold in favour of the receptor, whereas concentration of TeBG may be up to 30-fold higher than receptor concentrations. Methods proposed to solve this difficulty include the use of cultured skin fibroblasts (Keenan et al. 1974, 1975; Griffin et al. 1976; Kaufman et al. 1976), separation of the two proteins prior to receptor assay (Evain et al. 1977; Mowszowicz and Wright 1979), and the use of a synthetic ligand, methyltrienolone (R 1881), which binds to the androgen receptor and not to TeBG (Bonne et al. 1977; Menon et al. 1978). The principle for receptor assay in both cases is the same: parallel incubations are performed with the ^{3}H-ligand only (total binding), or the same concentration of the ^{3}H-ligand in presence of 100- to 500-fold excess of the same unlabeled molecule (non-specific binding). The difference yields the specific binding.

a) Cultured Fibroblasts

As already stated, fibroblasts were the first solution offered to eliminate the interference of TeBG. They also eliminate the problem of endogenous steroids, which in adult tissues, may occupy the binding sites. Binding measures can be performed on functionally intact cells, and the total receptor concentration (cytosol + nucleus) is usually measured. In addition, fibroblasts can be obtained from very small skin samples and they represent ideal tools for dynamic studies on the regulation of the androgen receptor.

However, successive subcultures result in clone heterogeneity in receptor concentration (Amrhein et al. 1976), which may lead to difficulties in appreciating the functional level of the androgen receptor in pathological conditions.

b) Cell-Free Extracts

Studies on cytosol of human skin have the advantage of being rapid and of assessing the actual receptor concentration at the time of sampling. They should be of great interest in clinical assessment of the androgen receptor. However, if the problem of TeBG can now be solved, there are other problems such as the occupancy of binding sites by endogenous steroids and the fact that, in the presence of endogenous hormones, most of the receptor is recovered in the nucleus (Menon et al. 1978). Thus, the assay of the cytosol receptor alone may be of little value. Most of our current knowledge on the androgen receptor, however, is still derived from studies of cultured fibroblasts.

2. Characterization of the Androgen Receptor

a) Physiochemical Properties

The androgen receptor of cultured skin fibroblasts sediments in sucrose gradient, as an 8 S protein at low salt concentration (Griffin et al. 1976), and as a 4 S protein at high salt concentration (Keenan et al. 1975). No direct information is currently available on the coefficient sedimentation of androgen in human skin cytosol. However, the androgen receptor of the rat prostate, which sediments as an 8 S protein, is eluted on sepharose column with the void volume, as is the androgen receptor of human skin (Mowszowicz and Wright 1979). A similar isoelectric point (5.2) has been reported in skin cytosol (Svensson and Snochowski 1979) and cytosol from human (Snochowski et al. 1978) and rat (Mainwaring and Irving 1973) prostate. Thus, in spite of the scarcity of data, it is not unreasonable to speculate that the androgen receptor from human skin has physiochemical characteristics very similar to those of the well-studied protein of the rat prostate.

b) Heat Lability

The extreme heat lability of the receptor in cell-free extracts is another characteristic of the androgen receptor of all tissues; binding activity is reduced to 20% of that of controls after a 1 h incubation at 20° C (Svensson and Snochowski 1979) and completely destroyed after 3 h at 15° C (Mowszowicz unpublished work). This raises methodological problems for the quantitative assay of binding capacity in human skin cytosol, as it prevents the use of classic exchange techniques to displace the endogenous steroids from binding sites.

c) Dissociation Constant

The androgen receptor of human skin has a high affinity for dihydrotestosterone ($K_D = 0.23 \pm 0.04 \cdot 10^{-9} M$) (Mowszowicz and Wright 1979) and for methyltrienolone ($K_D = 0.9 \pm 0.2 \cdot 10^{-9} M$) (Menon et al. 1978). Similar values have been found in cultured skin fibroblasts ($K_D = 0.1$ to $0.8 \cdot 10^{-9} M$) (Keenan et al. 1975; Lamberigts et al. 1979).

d) Specificity

The relative affinity of different steroids for the skin androgen receptor are as follows: dihydrotestosterone > testosterone > oestradiol > progesterone (Svensson and Snochowski 1979). Cortisol did not compete with dihydrotestosterone for binding sites. However, in a study using dihydrotestosterone as ligand, Rifka et al. (1978) reported no displacement of the binding by oestradiol or progesterone, but a 20% displacement by dexamethasone and a 50% displacement by spironolactones. In cultured skin fibroblasts, the apparent dissociation constant is similar for testosterone and dihydrotestosterone (Lamberigts et al. 1979; Maes et al. 1979).

The high affinity of the androgen receptor for testosterone is of particular interest. It has been shown that in target tissues deprived of 5α-reductase activity, such as the mouse kidney (Bardin et al. 1973), skeletal muscle (Michel and Baulieu 1975) or heart (Krieg et al. 1978), testosterone itself is the active androgen, i. e. binds to the androgen receptor and is transferred to the nucleus to promote androgen action. The same applies to the wolffian derivatives, in which 5α-reductase appears only after sexual differentiation (Siiteri and Wilson 1974). Patients with pseudohermaphroditism due to 5α-reductase deficiency, have normal levels of androgen receptor (Kuttenn et al. 1979 b; Maes et al. 1979); this could explain the virilization of their external genitalia at puberty with the increase of testosterone secretion.

3. Physiological Variations

Again, most of our knowledge is derived from cultured skin fibroblasts. Whereas the affinity of the androgen receptor is the same in all the areas studied (Keenan et al. 1975), confirming the unicity of this protein, its concentration varies with anatomical sites. The highest values are found in foreskin fibroblasts (about 1000

$\times 10^{-18}$ mol/µg DNA [Keenan et al. 1975]) which, assuming a mean DNA content of 10 pg per cell, represent around 15 000 binding sites per cell. However, normal values are widely scattered around this average value. In other territories tested (abdominal skin, neck skin, wrist) the concentration of androgen receptor is much less (100–200 $\times 10^{-18}$ mol/µg DNA). In contrast to 5α-reductase, neither sex differences for a given anatomical site nor variation with age has been observed (Griffin et al. 1976; Amrhein et al. 1977; Mowszowicz et al. 1979).

4. Control of Androgen Receptor Concentration

Nothing is yet known about the ontogenesis of the androgen receptor in the different territories where androgen action is essential for sexual differentiation. The question of its hormonal control also remains unanswered. However, the parity of values in men and women and the absence of variations with age, in parallel with changes of androgen secretion, argue against a regulation by androgen hormones of their own receptor. More work will be necessary to clarify this problem since the data in the literature on the hormonal control of the androgen receptor conflict. Thus, some authors have reported that in the rat prostate, or epididymis, the androgen receptor disappears after castration and can be restored by androgen treatment (Blondeau et al. 1975; Pujol and Bayard 1979), but others have denied this androgen dependence (Sullivan and Strott 1973; Calandra et al. 1977).

5. Pathological Variations

The importance of the androgen receptor is further emphasized by pathological models. The absence of the androgen receptor results in complete insensitivity to androgens, as in the complete form of testicular feminization syndrome. In incomplete forms of pseudohermaphroditism, decreased sensitivity has been related to decreased concentrations of the androgen receptor (Amrhein et al. 1977). There is only one report in the literature (Bonne et al. 1977) in which increased androgen action has been related to increased androgen receptor.

VI. Conclusion

Androgen action on its target cells depends on two factors: (1) the amount of available androgens provided through the blood stream, and (2) the capacity of target cells to utilize these androgens.

The amount of androgens provided through the blood depends on androgen secretion or blood production rates and on the extent of their binding to TeBG, which controls the entry in the target cell. The capacity of the target cell to utilize androgens rests on its ability to form dihydrotestosterone, the active androgen, from testosterone (5α-reduction) or from inactive precursors. It also requires the presence of a cytosolic receptor to bind dihydrotestosterone, transfer it to the nucleus, and promote specific androgen action.

Increased activity of the androgen target cell can result from one or both of the following mechanisms: increased production rate and/or increased utilization of available androgens by the target cell.

H. Clinical and Biological Assessment of Hirsutism

The clinical approach to hirsutism has two different aims:
1) To perform a correct evaluation of the degree of hirsutism and its eventual association to other clinical manifestations of abnormal androgenization, and
2) To obtain, by means of appropriate investigation, an indication of the aetiology of hirsutism in view of giving appropriate treatment.

I. Clinical Assessment

Considerable difficulties arise in the accurate assessment of the degree and severity of hirsutism in women. Different clinical methods have been proposed for evaluating the grading of terminal hair growth.
1. *The semi-quantitative method of Ferriman and Gallway* (1961), classifies hair growth by four categories of increasing severity in as many as eleven different sites in the body. The sum of the gradings provides an index of the overall severity of the condition (Table 4).
2. *A classification of hirsutism* among three degrees has been proposed by Abraham (1978):
a) *Slight:* small, pigmented hairs in one or several of the following localizations: lips and chin, but not extended to the whole beard area.
b) *Moderate:* coarse, large, strongly pigmented hair on the following sites: face, but not the whole beard area; chest, linea alba descending to the pubic area.
c) *Severe:* large pigmented hair on the whole beard territory.
3. *From a practical point of view*, hirsutism in women is essentially of three main types:
a) *With stigma of virilization* when progressive hair growth is associated with other clinical manifestations, notably a masculine contour, atrophy of the breasts, clitoral hypertrophy, male-type baldness, temporal recession and deepening of the voice.
b) *Without stigma of virilization* but associated with other pathological conditions such as seborrhoea, acne, menstrual disorders, enlarged ovaries on pelvic examination, and infertility.
c) *Idiopathic*, where no gross pathological defects are apparent.
4. *In our opinion* (Kuttenn and Mauvais-Jarvis 1978), the aetiology of hirsutism may be oriented by data obtained from clinical investigations (Table 5).

A recent and rapidly extensive hirsutism may be an indication of a virilizing tumour, particularly of adrenal origin.

Hirsutism which appears at the onset of puberty, accompanied by a progressive oligomenorrhoea or amenorrhoea and enlarged ovaries, is probably due to a polycystic ovary syndrome.

Table 4. Hair gradings according to Ferriman and Gallway (1961)

Site	Grade	Definition
Upper lip	1	A few hairs at outer margin
	2	A small moustache at outer margin
	3	A moustache extending halfway from outer margin
	4	A moustache extending to mid-line
Chin	1	A few scattered hairs
	2	Scattered hairs with small concentrations
	3, 4	Complete cover, light and heavy
Chest	1	Circumareolar hairs
	2	With mid-line hair in addition
	3	Fusion of these areas, with three-quarter cover
	4	Complete cover
Upper back	1	A few scattered hairs
	2	Rather more still scattered
	3, 4	Complete cover, light and heavy
Lower back	1	A sacral tuft of hair
	2	With some lateral extension
	3	Three-quarter cover
	4	Complete cover
Upper abdomen	1	A few mid-line hairs
	2	Rather more, still mid-line
	3, 4	Half and full cover
Lower abdomen	1	A few mid-line hairs
	2	A mid-line streak of hair
	3	A mid-line band of hair
	4	An inverted V-shaped growth
Arm	1	Sparse growth affecting not more than a quarter of the limb surface
	2	More than this; cover still incomplete
	3, 4	Complete cover, light and heavy
Forearm	1–4	Complete cover of dorsal surface; 2 grades of light and 2 of heavy growth
Thigh	1–4	As for arm
Leg	1–4	As for forearm

Table 5. Relationship between clinical features and expected diagnosis in hirsutism

Clinical findings relative to hirsutism	Expected diagnosis
Recent, explosive, clitoromegaly	Tumour (ovarian or adrenal)
Onset at puberty, menstrual disorders	Polycystic ovary syndrome
Associated with virilization of external genitalia	
Increased muscle mass	Delayed onset congenital
Short stature	adrenal hyperplasia
Delayed menarche	
Familial history	
Onset at puberty, no menstrual disorder, no virilization Familial history, ethnic origin	Idiopathic hirsutism

An old and marked hirsutism with partial virilization of the external genitalia, even restricted to clitoromegaly with male morphology, short stature, delayed menarche and familial antecedents, is in favour of an adrenal origin, particularly a delayed onset of adrenal hyperplasia.

An ancient and moderate hirsutism, generalized but with seborrhoea and acne, progressively extended with familial or ethnic characteristics, is probably related to "idiopathic hirsutism" with increased end organ sensitivity and no hypersecretion of active androgen by ovaries or adrenals.

II. Hormonal Investigation of Hirsutism

It must be emphasized that hirsutism should not be regarded as a static condition confined to a specific organ, but rather as a disorder in which changes in the functional integrity of a number of organs may occur concomitantly. Thus, although excessive hair growth may be initiated by a specific defect in one endocrine gland, subsequent changes in the function of other endocrine parameters, i.e. liver and skin, are likely to occur and influence the general picture.

Historically, two different periods must be considered regarding the hormonal investigation of hirsutism. The first period is essentially concerned with the determination of urinary 17-ketosteroids and other metabolites of secreted precursors, in particular, pregnanetriol and 17-hydrocorticosteroids. The second period is directly issued from the development of reliable plasma assays for circulating androgens.

1. Urinary 17-Ketosteroids

a) Basal Conditions

Urinary 17-ketosteroids in women are generally believed to originate from precursors secreted mainly by the adrenal cortex and the ovary. Two important 17-ketosteroids derived from testosterone and androstenedione are androsterone, which possesses androgenic potency, and etiocholanolone, which is inert. Both compounds are also derived from other precursors of varying androgenic potencies. Urinary dehydroisoandrosterone determination has been proposed for the evaluation of hirsutism of adrenal origin (Abraham 1978). In fact, dehydroisoandrosterone is not an active androgen and it has not been proven that the hypersecretion of this steroid may be responsible for the development of hirsutism (Mauvais-Jarvis and Kuttenn 1976).

The main advantage of measuring 17-ketosteroids, especially in urine, lies in the fact that available techniques are simple and rapid, being ideally suited for use in routine laboratories. By the estimation of 17-ketosteroids in urine, it is generally possible to differentiate hirsutism arising from major adrenal disease from that resulting from ovarian disease. In the former type, significantly high 17-ketosteroid levels are found, whereas in the latter, readings are usually within the normal range.

The main limitation of 17-ketosteroid assays is that such estimations do not provide a precise index of androgenic function, there being a considerable overlap between values found in normal men and women. Furthermore, it is possible for a potent androgen such as testosterone to be produced in the body in excessive amounts without this fact being mirrored in the levels of 17-ketosteroids in blood or urine. This presumably explains the well-documented findings that in many patients with idiopathic hirsutism, measurements of total or fractionated 17-ketosteroids in urine are within the normal range.

b) Tests of Ovarian Function

In order to localize the site of excessive androgen production, several dynamic tests have been proposed.

In hirsute women, the ovarian contribution to the androgen pool has been determined following stimulation with HCG and suppression by the use of oestrogens or progestogen-oestrogen mixtures (generally administered in the form of an oral contraceptive) (Wieland et al. 1967; Lloyd 1966; Lloyd et al. 1966; Ismael and Loraine 1969; Maroulis et al. 1977). In some reports (Jayle et al. 1962; Jayle 1967), an ovarian stimulation test was conducted concomitantly with an adrenal suppression test using dexamethasone. It should be emphasized that the compounds administered, the dosage and duration of therapy, and the clinical design of the investigation varied greatly in the hands of different workers (Ismael and Loraine 1969). On the basis of such studies, it has been claimed that an ovarian component in the pathogenesis of hirsutism can be recognized. This may well be so, but it must be pointed out that the tests used to substantiate this hypothesis do not appear to have been completely reliable. Indeed, in polycystic ovary type I (Stein-Leventhal syndrome), the pituitary secretion of LH being already elevated, the ovarian secretion of androgen may not increase after HCG administration. In that case the urinary excretion of androsterone and etiocholanolone is not modified by the test. The same test, using the simultaneous administration of HCG and dexamethasone, is very difficult to interpret since dexamethasone not only inhibits secretion of ACTH and the adrenal, but also the biosynthesis of gonadal androgens (Evain et al. 1976). This may also explain the results observed by Kirschner et al. (1966 b) in idiopathic hirsutism. These authors showed that dexamethasone decreased plasma testosterone and androstenedione in hirsute patients in whom catheterization findings strongly suggested the ovaries as the source of these androgens.

c) Tests of Adrenal Function

Androgen production by the adrenal cortex is generally assessed by administration of ACTH for purposes of stimulation and by the administration of a variety of potent corticosteroids for purposes of suppression (Lloyd 1966; Lloyd et al. 1966; Maroulis et al. 1977; Givens 1976).

As with tests involving the ovary, the type of investigation conducted and the material administered varied greatly from one investigator to another. Thus, in the case of ACTH, intramuscular and subcutaneous injections were given, and the hormone was administered in widely varying dosages, commonly as a gel or zinc. The most frequently used corticosteroid has undoubtedly been dexamethasone, but prednisone and prednisolone have been employed in addition.

Techniques for the assessment of adrenocortical function in hirsute patients have proved useful but are not completely reliable. For example, in some women, in whom hirsutism was associated with polycystic ovaries and not with manifest adrenal disease, a marked decrease in androgen levels occurred following a suppression test with dexamethasone (Horton and Neilser 1968). In addition, during stimulation tests with ACTH, plasma and urinary testosterone levels and testosterone production rates in hirsute patients with polycystic ovaries have been shown to vary greatly, increasing in some or decreasing in others (Shearman and Cox 1966).

2. Plasma Androgens

a) Assays of Testosterone

Methods for determining testosterone in plasma and biological fluids have evolved over the past decade from time-consuming double isotope approach methods, electron-capture gas chromatography or competitive protein binding, to present-day methods using essentially radioimmunoassay approaches. These methods are far simpler and more accurate than earlier methods. In addition, radioimmunoassay can be set up in any endocrinological laboratory.

α) *Urinary Testosterone Excretion.* Of the testosterone production rate only 1% is excreted in urine as testosterone glucuronide (Camacho and Migeon 1963). Normal women excrete approximately 4 µg testosterone glucuronide per 24 h, more than twice than expected from a plasma production rate of 230 µg/24 h. The apparent discrepancy between plasma and urinary testosterone is explained by the observation that plasma steroids, other than testosterone, serve as precursors of testosterone glucuronide. In the liver and other sites (the skin, for instance) androstenedione and dehydroisoandrosterone are converted to testosterone which is then conjugated to glucuronic acid before entering the plasma testosterone pool. Urinary testosterone in women, therefore, does not accurately reflect the plasma testosterone production rate (Kirschner and Bardin 1972).

β) *Plasma Testosterone* (Fig. 12) (Table 1). The mean plasma testosterone level for normal women is 0.35 ng/ml (range 0.20–0.45 ng/ml); although a small circadian rhythm of plasma testosterone is synchronous with that of cortisol in normal women, it is not statistically significant (James et al. 1976). Givens (1976) found that variation in plasma testosterone of 11 normal women throughout a 24 h period were only 0.11 ± 0.03 ng/ml. Consequently, the time of day at which blood is drawn is not so important in evaluating plasma testosterone value. However, the proper interpretation of a given plasma testosterone value does require knowledge of the plasma TeBG binding capacity, since the largest fraction of plasma testosterone is bound. A normal plasma testosterone value, with an abnormally lower TeBG binding capacity, suggests a possible increase in circulating free and biologically active testosterone. Exogenous oestrogens and pregnancy increase the TeBG binding capacity (Vermeulen et al. 1969). On the other hand, in women it is decreased by testosterone treatment and is generally low in hirsute females (Vermeulen et al. 1969; Dray et al. 1968a). So, methods have been devised to quantify free testosterone and total plasma androgens in an effort to circumvent these difficulties, but the general usefulness of these parameters remains to be established (Rosenfield 1971; Vermeulen et al. 1971).

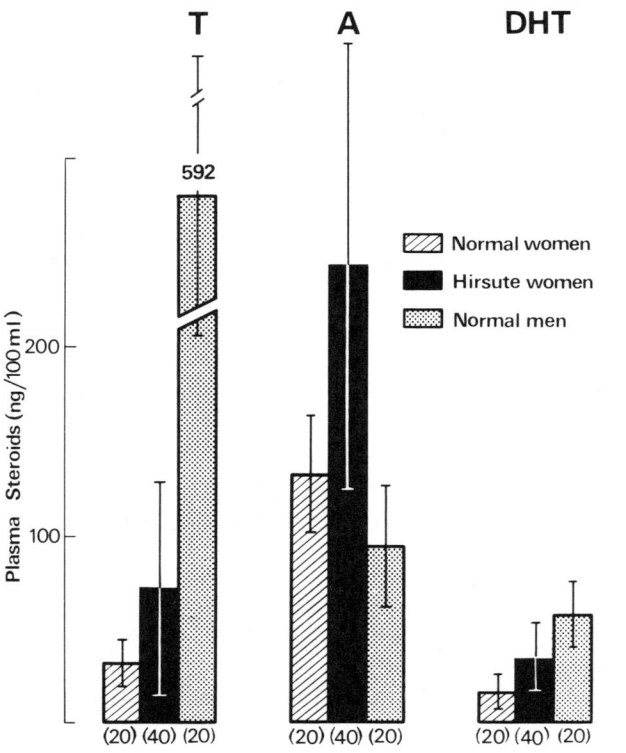

Fig. 12. Plasma testosterone (*T*), androstenedione (*A*) and dihydrotestosterone (*DHT*) in 20 normal men, 20 normal women and 40 women with hirsutism of various origins

γ) *Testosterone Production Rate.* Testosterone production rates were first estimated by Korenman et al. (1963), using the urinary isotope dilution principle, and values of 7 mg/day for normal men seemed perfectly reasonable. However, when this method was used to assess testosterone production in women, values of 1–2 mg/day seemed unreasonably high. Subsequent studies by these workers (Korenman and Lipsett 1964) demonstrated that the isolated urinary testosterone glucuronide was not a unique metabolite of plasma testosterone; and at lower levels of androgen production (in normal and virilized women) prehormones can be converted directly to testosterone glucuronide, leading to three- or fourfold overestimation of testosterone production rates. To determine metabolic clearance rates, Tait and Horton (1966) developed the constant infusion approach which provided a way to measure hormone production rates, without having to rely on urinary metabolites. The product of plasma hormone concentration and its metabolic clearance rate equals the blood production rate of the hormone, or the amount of hormone that enters the blood from all sources per unit time. By this technique the testosterone production rate in normal women is 230 ± 73 µg/day. The production rate is perhaps the most accurate determination for the physician as it correlates better with virilization than any other measure of androgen determination. Even though the production rate may be the best test, it is not necessarily the most practical for extensive clinical use, as it requires independent determination of the plasma testosterone concentration and the metabolic clearance rate. Although plasma testosterone can now be easily determined, estimation of the metabolic clearance

Table 6. Results obtained by different authors from the evaluation of testosterone in biological fluids in normal and hirsute women (range)

	Normal women	Hirsute women
Plasma testosterone concentration (ng/ml)	0.2–0.4	0.3–5.0
Plasma free testosterone (pg/ml)	1.5–10.0	4.3–50.0
Testosterone blood production rate (µg/24 h)	130–330	550–2640
Metabolic clearance rate (1/24 h)	530–760	590–1750

rate requires multiple blood samples during constant infusion of radioactive testosterone (Kirschner and Bardin 1972) (Table 6).

b) Assays of Androstenedione

Androstenedione is a particularly important parameter since up to 50% of the blood production rate of testosterone in women is contributed by this steroid (Horton and Tait 1966). In addition, most of the dihydrotestosterone originates from androstenedione (Ito and Horton 1971) and for Vermeulen and Ando (1979), the larger fraction of intracellular dihydrotestosterone in women comes from plasma androstenedione. As neither intracellular testosterone nor dihydrotestosterone are necessarily end metabolites secreted into the plasma (Wright et al. 1978), high androgen levels in peripheral tissues should not necessarily show up in plasma as testosterone and dihydrotestosterone.

In normal adult women, androstenedione is secreted equally by both adrenals and ovaries. Moreover, since androstenedione is not bound to a specific protein, and since the metabolic clearance rate of this steroid is reported to be normal in hirsute patients (Bardin and Lipsett 1967), the plasma levels reflect androstenedione production more accurately than testosterone levels reflect testosterone production. However, changes in plasma androstenedione levels occur through the menstrual cycle. The concentration of androstenedione in the early follicular phase of the cycle is below the normal range for women, but rises twofold towards midcycle (Baird 1976). Thus in hirsute patients with ovulatory cycles, blood samples for androstenedione determination must be obtained during the follicular phase or after ovulation. In spite of these restrictions, the determination of androstenedione in the plasma of hirsute women is certainly an essential step in hormonal investigation (Fig. 12).

c) Dynamic Tests for Plasma Testosterone and Androstenedione

As for urinary 17-ketosteroids, the determination of plasma testosterone during stimulation tests (using ACTH or HCG) and suppression tests (using dexamethasone or oestrogens) failed to give useful information that might aid the clinician in localizing the origin of excessive androgen production. Indeed, plasma testosterone in normal and hirsute women decreases during glucocorticoid administration due to the fact that cortisol and gonadal corticosteroids may interfere with receptors for LH (Evain et al. 1976). This may explain why plasma testosterone and androstenedione decrease after dexamethasone administration in hirsutism of both adrenal and ovarian origin (Fig. 13). For the same reasons, ACTH,

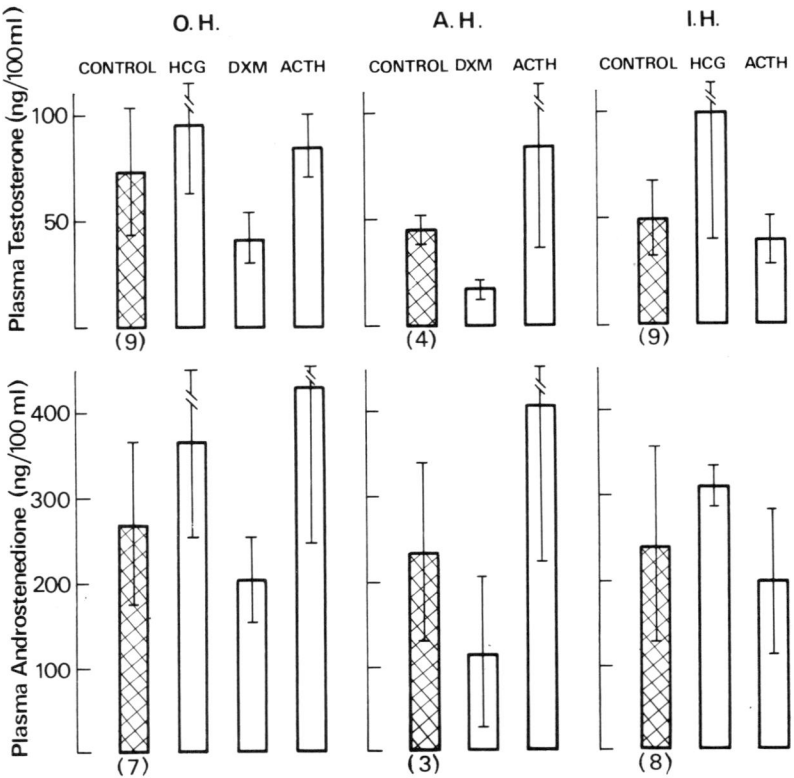

Fig. 13. Plasma testosterone and androstenedione in hirsute women during dynamic tests. *HCG*, 15 000 IU chorionic gonadotropins. *DXM*, 2.5 mg daily × 5 days dexamethasone; *ACTH*, 250 µg synthetic ACTH; *O.H.*, hirsutism of ovarian origin; *A.H.*, hirsutism of adrenal origin; *I.H.*, idiopathic hirsutism

when injected in women with idiopathic hirsutism, decreases both plasma testosterone and androstenedione (Fig. 14).

Finally, the usefulness of oestrogen suppression in localizing the site of androgen production is difficult to support because oestrogen treatment produces a 50% decrease of testosterone metabolic clearance rate. In hirsutism of ovarian origin, however, HCG administration is generally responsible for a significant increase in plasma testosterone and androstenedione (Fig. 13).

d) Ovarian and Adrenal Vein Catheterization

In view of the inadequacies of other tests in localizing the sites of androgen production in hirsute women, selective catheterization of ovarian and adrenal veins has been developed. These studies can be accomplished on conscious patients and provide not only blood samples for hormonal analysis, but also X-ray visualization by means of reflux venography. There are many problems associated with the catheterization approach. Technically, these are difficult vessels to locate in view of their size and unpredictable location. Blood flow from these vessels is often quite slow and the vessels tend easily to go into spasm during the sampling procedure. Both adrenal and ovarian veins are diluted in their course with phrenic and lumbar

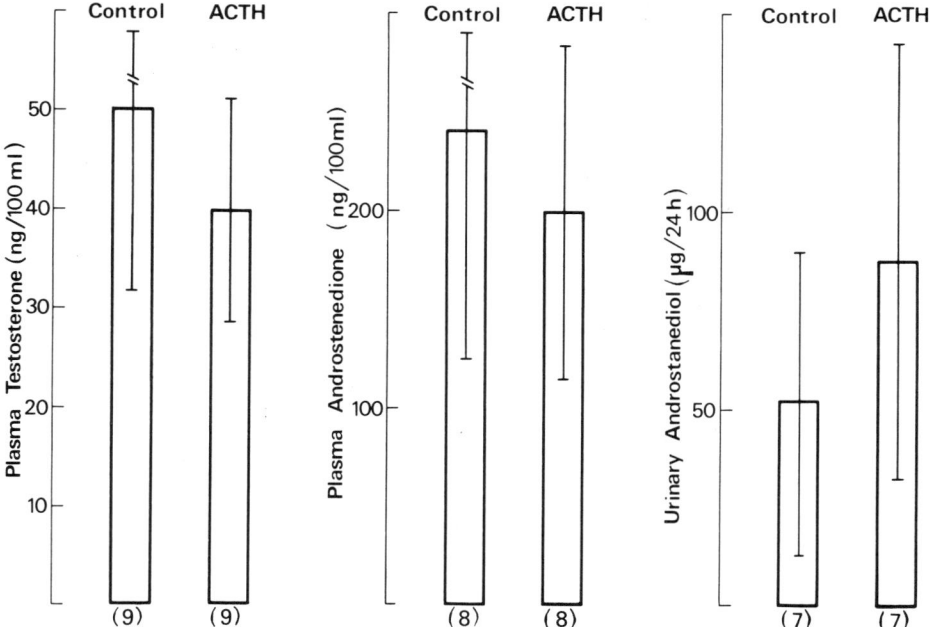

Fig. 14. Plasma testosterone and androstenedione, urinary androstanediol before and after 250 µg synthetic ACTH injected into women with idiopathic hirsutism

vessels, respectively. Kirschner and co-workers (1976a) postulated that venous catheterization, in spite of important technical difficulties, offers the best and most direct approach to determining the sites of overproduction in women with documented hirsutism. This method seems particularly indicated for the diagnosis and localization of ovarian and adrenal tumours (Kirschner and Jacobs 1971).

e) Dihydrotestosterone

Plasma dihydrotestosterone does not arise from direct secretion, but essentially reflects events occurring in peripheral target tissues. In men, the major precursor of plasma dihydrotestosterone is testosterone. In women, androstenedione appears to be the major precursor of plasma dihydrotestosterone (Ito and Horton 1971). However, in hirsutism, dihydrotestosterone levels are not significantly elevated. This may reflect altered binding to plasma TeBG, as well as the fact that most of dihydrotestosterone synthesized in target tissues (particularly the skin) is reduced in situ to 3α- and 3β-androstanediols, whereas only a small fraction of dihydrotestosterone enters the blood (Kuttenn et al. 1977).

f) Other Steroids

The determination of plasma dehydroisoandrosterone and particularly of dehydroisoandrosterone sulphate may be interesting for evaluating the androgen function of the adrenal cortex. In most cases of hirsutism, the amount of these two androgens is within the normal range except in the case of adrenal tumours. It may be difficult to interpret the plasma values of dehydroisoandrosterone, since they fluctuate, in parallel with cortisol levels, suggesting ACTH-dependent secretion.

Plasma dehydroisoandrosterone sulphate does not because of the long half-life of this steroid (James et al. 1976).

The plasma determination of 17α-hydroprogesterone is very useful, particularly after ACTH stimulation in hirsute patients with a clinical history evoking a delayed onset of adrenal hyperplasia.

3. Evaluation of Androstanediols

In target cells, most of the dihydrotestosterone is converted to 3α- and 3β-androstanediols. In addition, plasma dihydrotestosterone is converted to a greater extent to 3α- rather than 3β-diol (Mahoudeau et al. 1971), whereas circulating 3β-androstanediol is largely converted into 3α-androstanediol, which is excreted in the urine (Mauvais-Jarvis et al. 1970 b). Thus the determination of 3α-androstanediol in biological fluids is very useful for the hormonal assessment of hirsutism. In our opinion, the determination of 3α-androstanediol in the urine gives more useful information than the plasma assay of this steroid (Kuttenn et al. 1977; Wright et al. 1978). This assumption is substantiated by the fact that the estimation rate of 3α-androstanediol production in blood (Mahoudeau et al. 1971; Kinouchi and Horton 1974) is similar to the daily excretion rates. However, plasma radioimmunoassay of 3α-androstanediol has been proposed for the clinical investigation of hirsutism (Habrioux et al. 1978). From a physiological point of view, the major source of 3α-androstanediol in men is testosterone. The production of this androgen in this sex

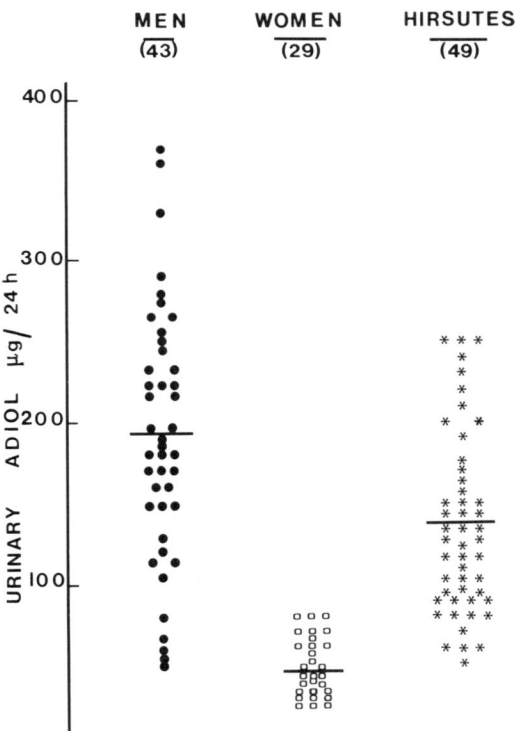

Fig. 15. Urinary 3α-androstanediol (*Adiol*) excretion in normal men, women and women with hirsutism of various origins. Wright et al. 1978

Table 7. Theoretical contribution to urinary Adiol of secreted androgens: testosterone (T); androstenedione (Δ_4); dehydroisoandrosterone (D); dehydroisoandrosterone sulfate (DS); in normal adult subjects (range)

Precursors	Conversion rate of secreted androgens to urinary Adiol[a]		Expected urinary Adiol excretion[b]	
	Men (%)	Women (%)	Men µg/24 h	Women µg/24 h
T	1.0–2.5	0.4–0.5	50–250	5–10
Δ_4	0.5–1.0	0.4–0.5	10– 20	15–20
D+DS	0.1	0.1	10– 30	10–20
SUM			70–300	30–50

[a] Percent conversion to urinary adiol of radioactive androgens injected intravenously (Mauvais-Jarvis et al. 1968).
[b] Calculated from conversion rate of secreted androgens to urinary adiol and blood production rate of androgens in normal individuals.

depends not only on gonadal secretion, but also on variations in 5α-reductase activity (Kuttenn et al. 1975, 1977). This may explain the wide range of urinary 3α-androstanediol observed in normal men (Fig. 15).

In women, 3α-androstanediol mainly originates from the conversion of androstenedione to testosterone and dihydrotestosterone. The variations in androstenedione production during the menstrual cycle are not sufficient to modify significantly the 3α-androstanediol excretion. In hirsute women, the increase of both androstenedione production and skin metabolism may account for the striking difference in 3α-androstanediol urinary excretion observed between these patients and normal women (Mauvais-Jarvis et al. 1973). The contribution of testosterone in the blood to the level of 3α-androstanediol in the urine of hirsute patients leads to the conclusion that, at most, 20 µg of the urinary 3α-androstanediol excreted per 24 h could arise from testosterone (Table 7). The contribution of plasma dehydroisoandrosterone and dehydroisoandrosterone sulphate to urinary 3α-androstanediol is low and identical in both sexes: at most, 30 µg per 24 h. In other words, variations of androstenedione production and skin "utilization" may account for a daily excretion of 3α-androstanediol which ranges from 12 to 100 µg/24 h (Kuttenn et al. 1977; Mauvais-Jarvis et al. 1973; Wright et al. 1978).

4. Conclusion

The assessment of hirsutism in women involves, first, an adequate evaluation of the clinical findings, regarding particularly the mode of evolution of the disease, its eventual association with other symptoms of virilization and/or the possible existence of menstrual abnormalities. The determination of the plasma testosterone level gives the most useful information concerning the seriousness of the disease. When plasma testosterone remains below 1.0 ng/ml, hirsutism is likely due to a functional abnormality in the secretion of endocrine glands and/or the skin "utilization" of androgens. In that case, the determination of plasma androstenedione and urinary 3α-androstanediol may give very important information regarding the respective participation of the overproduction of androgens and their end-organ utilization.

By contrast, if plasma testosterone is above 2.0 ng/ml, the diagnosis of virilizing tumour or congenital adrenal hyperplasia may be evoked. The simultaneous determination of plasma androstenedione is important to know whether testosterone is secreted by itself or if this plasma level essentially derives from the conversion of a high level of secreted androstenedione. In our opinion, except in certain limited cases, the dynamic tests cannot give very accurate information concerning the origin of such hypersecretion of androgen. In spite of important technical difficulties, venous catheterization is, from a theoretical point of view, the only method permitting an accurate localization of virilizing tumours originating from the adrenals and particularly the ovaries (Fig. 16).

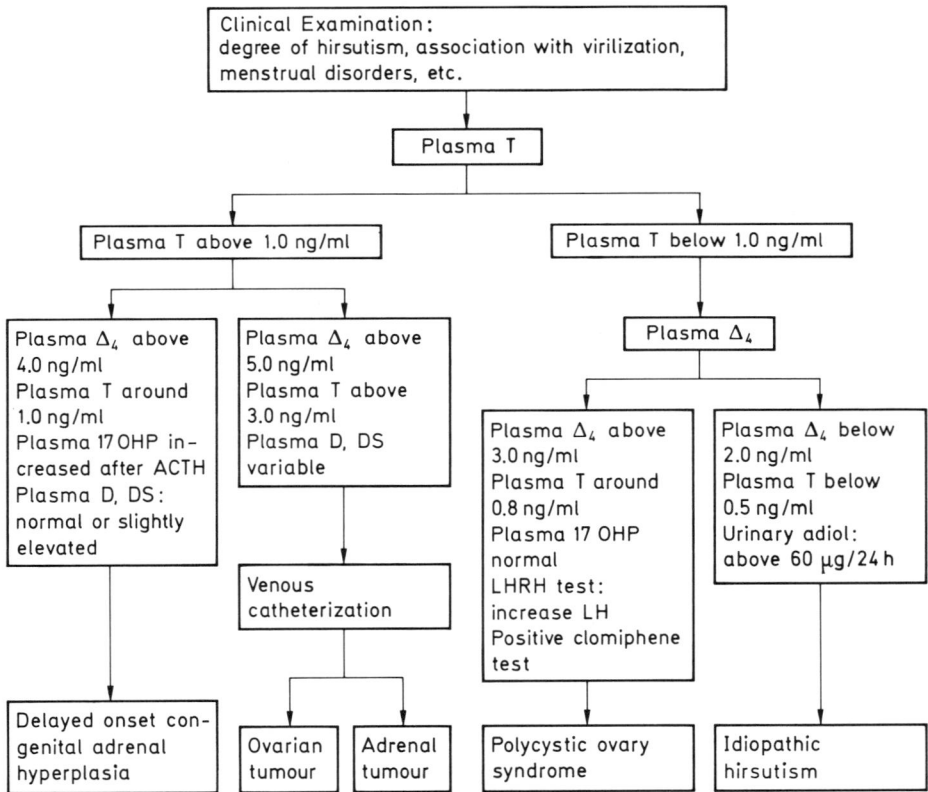

Fig. 16. A schematic guide for clinical and hormonal investigation of hirsute women. *T*, testosterone *Δ₄*, androstenedione; *D*, dehydroisoandrosterone; *DS*, dehydroisoandrosterone sulphate; *17 OHP*, 17α-hydroxyprogesterone

I. Hirsutism of Adrenal Origin

The role of an oversecretion of active androgens by adrenals in the development of hirsutism is controversial, particularly in the case of polycystic ovarian syndrome and idiopathic hirsutism (see Sects. J.I, K.). However, the only unquestionable aspects of adrenal virilism are represented by congenital adrenal hyperplasia due to enzymatic defects and by virilizing tumours of the adrenals.

I. Congenital Adrenal Hyperplasia Due to 21-Hydroxylase Deficiency

1. Introduction

Most of the reports concerning virilizing syndromes due to enzymatic defect of adrenal steroidogenesis have been described in female pseudohermaphroditism. In these cases, the clinical features of the disease are congenital or become apparent in infancy or in childhood. However, delayed onset of virilization in adult ages has been reported in subjects whose hormonal patterns were close to those found in congenital adrenal hyperplasia. Decourt et al. (1957) and Jayle et al. (1958) have observed several girls with normal external genitalia who developed virilization at puberty. They had hormonal abnormalities characteristic of the congenital disorder. Brooks et al. (1960) reported three similar cases in girls after the menarche. The similarity in response to cortisone therapy of patients with female pseudohermaphroditism due to congenital adrenal hyperplasia and patients having only acquired hirsutism, menstrual abnormalities and slightly elevated urinary 17-ketosteroids, led Jones et al. (1953, 1954) to suggest that this group of patients could have a mild form of congenital virilizing adrenal hyperplasia.

Congenital adrenal hyperplasia is due to 21-hydroxylase deficiency in approximately 95% of cases (New 1968). It is now well established that congenital adrenal hyperplasia due to 21-hydroxylase defect can manifest itself with various degrees of severity, one extreme being the salt-losing form, the other the mild, non-salt-losing form. The delayed onset form of congenital adrenal hyperplasia could represent an even milder or attenuated form of this syndrome without masculinization of the external genitalia of the females during fetal life, and mild adrenal hyperfunction after puberty. Whether such patients represent an acquired form of congenital adrenal hyperplasia or a group in which the clinical manifestations of the congenital form are delayed, has long remained controversial. By utilizing recently described methods for detection of the heterozygote carriers of congenital adrenal hyperplasia, Gutai et al. (1977) suggested that the so-called delayed onset congenital adrenal hyperplasia was an attenuated form of an homozygous state of congenital adrenal hyperplasia.

This "adult onset" and mild form of congenital adrenal hyperplasia should be considered in the different diagnosis of idiopathic hirsutism. Although it is a rare cause of hirsutism, it is readily treatable, and an effort should therefore be made to do so.

2. Frequency

Congenital adrenal hyperplasia due to 21-hydroxylase deficiency is an autosomal recessive disorder (Childs et al. 1956). The incidence of this disease in the white population is about 1:7000 (Prader 1958; Mauthe et al. 1977). Based upon this ratio, the frequency of heterozygous carriers has been calculated to be about 1:40.

3. Pathophysiology

a) General Remarks

21-Hydroxylation steps occur in the biosynthetic pathway of major steroids secreted by adrenal glands, i.e. cortisol and aldosterone. Cortisol biosynthesis takes place in the zona fasciculata through two successive steps: (1) a 21-hydroxylation of 17-hydroxyprogesterone into 11-deoxycortisol; and (2) an 11-hydroxylation of 11-deoxycortisol into cortisol. Aldosterone is synthesized in the zona glumerulosa from progesterone through the same hydroxylation steps (Table 8).

An adrenal 21-hydroxylase deficiency is responsible for a defect in glucocorticoid secretion (Bongiovanni and Root 1963; Bongiovanni et al. 1967) and, to a lesser extent, for a defect in mineralocorticoid secretion. The subsequent overstimulation of adrenals by ACTH is in turn responsible for an excessive synthesis of 17-hydroxyprogesterone, the steroid precursor immediately before the 21-hydroxy-

Table 8. Biosynthetic pathways for adrenal steroids

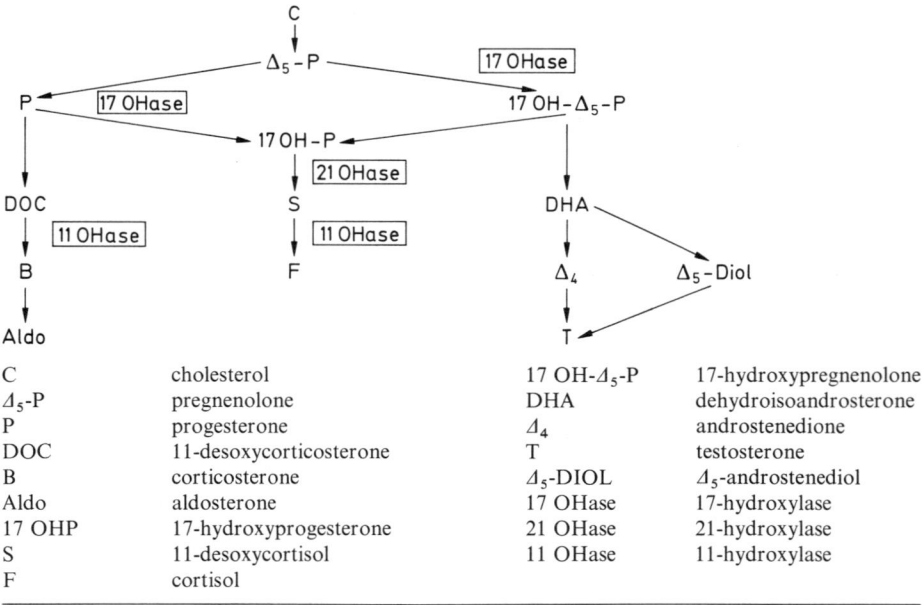

C	cholesterol	17 OH-Δ_5-P		17-hydroxypregnenolone
Δ_5-P	pregnenolone	DHA		dehydroisoandrosterone
P	progesterone	Δ_4		androstenedione
DOC	11-desoxycorticosterone	T		testosterone
B	corticosterone	Δ_5-DIOL		Δ_5-androstenediol
Aldo	aldosterone	17 OHase		17-hydroxylase
17 OHP	17-hydroxyprogesterone	21 OHase		21-hydroxylase
S	11-desoxycortisol	11 OHase		11-hydroxylase
F	cortisol			

lation in the cortisol biosynthetic pathway. In addition there is an overproduction of adrenal androgens for which 17-hydroxyprogesterone is also a precursor.

In so far as congenital adrenal hyperplasia due to 21-hydroxylase deficiency is concerned, certain definitions are necessary, since several terms are used to distinguish salt-losing or non-salt-losing forms, complete or partial enzymatic defects and also delayed or acquired forms of the disease. In all cases, however, biological data prove a defect in 21-hydroxylase enzyme activity. This defect expresses itself in a wide variety of manifestations such as: (1) salt-losing syndrome, (2) virilization of the external genitalia at birth, or (3) delayed onset virilization.

In the case of complete enzyme defect, earlier clinical symptoms occur, in particular the salt-losing syndrome and major virilization resulting from an insufficiency in both cortisol and aldosterone secretion and from an adrenal androgen overproduction. In the case of partial defect, the deficiency only occurs in the glucocorticoid pathway. It may only be expressed by an androgen overproduction, the intensity and delayed onset of which depend upon the severity of the enzyme defect.

b) Single or Multiple Enzymes

Patients with salt-losing congenital adrenal hyperplasia are unable to produce sufficient amounts of cortisol and aldosterone. In non-salt-losing patients, only cortisol production seems to be impaired (Kowarski et al. 1965; Bartter et al. 1968; Degenhart et al. 1965). Since 21-hydroxylation is defective in both forms of congenital adrenal hyperplasia, and since the enzyme is required for the biosynthesis of both cortisol and aldosterone, the different aspects of steroid deficiency are difficult to interpret. Two theories have been proposed: a "single enzyme" theory (Bongiovanni 1958) and a "multiple enzyme" theory (Bryan et al. 1965; West et al. 1979). According to the single enzyme theory, there is a single 21-hydroxylase system for both cortisol and aldosterone biosynthesis. In non-salt-losers the enzymatic defect could be partial and mild. Steroid precursors of cortisol biosynthesis should be diverted into the aldosterone pathway in a sufficient concentration to overcome the enzymatic defect in aldosterone biosynthesis, particularly since daily needs and production of aldosterone are normally 150 times lesser than cortisol production. The enzymatic defect could be too severe in salt-losing patients to be overcome by this compensatory mechanism; thus, a decrease in aldosterone production might occur.

In the multiple enzyme theory, it is hypothesized that there are two separate and different 21-hydroxylase systems for cortisol and aldosterone biosynthesis. According to this theory, salt-losing patients would have an inherited defect in both enzymes, while in non-salt-losers, only the enzyme specific for cortisol biosynthesis could be defective.

4. Androgen Production in 21-Hydroxylase Deficiency

Most studies on androgen production and interconversion in congenital adrenal hyperplasia due to 21-hydroxylase deficiency concern the complete form of the syndrome. Only a few studies have investigated the delayed onset forms of the disease. The overproduction of androgen in 21-hydroxylase deficiency essentially depends on the hypersecretion of ACTH due to the absence of cortisol negative feedback on the hypothalamus and the pituitary. Consequently, 17-hydroxyprogesterone production is increased and its level depends on the partial or complete character of the block (Strott et al. 1969; Franks 1974; Gourmelen et al. 1979). Progesterone production is also increased but its level is higher in the salt-losing form of 21-hydroxylase deficiency than in the non-salt-losing form (Strott et al. 1969).

In contrast, Δ_5-3β-hydroxysteroids are only slightly elevated: 1.5–2.0 times the normal level, with considerable overlapping with normal subjects (Loriaux et al. 1974). The moderate increase in (Δ_5-3β-hydroxysteroid secretion contrasting with the important Δ_4-steroid production suggests that under ACTH stimulation steroidogenesis is directed towards the Δ_4-pathway. Studies have been carried out to ascertain which Δ_4 androgens are secreted and which are responsible for virilization. Plasma androstenedione concentration is found to be six to seven times higher than normal (Horton and Frasier 1967; Rivarola et al. 1967c). This androstenedione production originates from a direct adrenal secretion and from the peripheral conversion of precursors. Dehydroisoandrosterone and Δ_5-androstenediol are not produced in sufficient amounts to contribute significantly to plasma androstenedione. In contrast, 17-hydroxyprogesterone, largely secreted by the adrenals, may be peripherally converted into androstenedione (Loriaux et al. 1974).

A direct testosterone secretion by the adrenals has been hypothesized from the observation of an increased testosterone urinary excretion (Camacho and Migeon 1963, 1966; Futterweit et al. 1965) and an increased testosterone plasma concentration and blood production rate (Korenman et al. 1965; Coppage and Cooner 1965). However, two-thirds of blood testosterone in the normal female are derived from blood androstenedione (Horton and Tait 1966). Horton and Frasier (1967) calculated that almost all the testosterone production of patients with congenital adrenal hyperplasia is derived from blood androstenedione. Thus, a direct adrenal secretion of testosterone is probably minimal in this disease.

5. Clinical and Hormonal Characteristics of Delayed Onset Congenital Adrenal Hyperplasia Due to 21-Hydroxylase Deficiency

From a clinical point of view, the so-called adult onset, mild form of congenital adrenal hyperplasia due to partial 21-hydroxylase deficiency is difficult to distinguish from hirsutism of other origins, particularly from idiopathic hirsutism. Some patients are observed for sterility, but they generally complain of acquired, postpubertal hirsutism with no other symptoms of virilization except, in rare cases, a certain degree of clitoromegaly. They are of normal weight, sometimes of a relatively short stature. They had a normal puberty and their menstrual cycles are normal and ovulatory.

a) Hormonal Data from the Literature

The diagnosis of 21-hydroxylase deficiency essentially depends on the biochemical evidence of the enzymatic deficiency. Of particular interest is the observation of a plasma level of 17-hydroxyprogesterone 50–200 times higher than normal (Strott et al. 1969) associated with an increase in the production of adrenal androgens. In fact, the diagnosis of partial defect in 21-hydroxylase has long been based on the observation of an elevated urinary excretion of pregnanetriol, the metabolite of 17-hydroxyprogesterone and of 17-ketosteroids (Decourt et al. 1957; Jayle et al. 1958).

This methodology does not seem to be actually accurate. Plasma 17-hydroxyprogesterone assay provides a more sensitive and convenient index of the enzymatic defect. However, in partial 21-hydroxylase defect, baseline levels of plasma 17-hydroxyprogesterone are generally only slightly above normal levels. This aspect is quite different from that observed in patients with a complete defect in whom plasma 17-hydroxyprogesterone is elevated even in basal conditions (Barnes and Atherden 1972; Pham-Huu-Trung et al. 1973; Franks 1974; Hughes and Winter 1976).

In patients with partial enzymatic defect, plasma cortisol may be low, but it is often normal. Plasma ACTH should be elevated as in the complete form of this syndrome. In fact, it is usually found to be within the normal range. Thus, dynamic tests using stimulation by ACTH are generally necessary to detect a partial defect in 21-hydroxylase (Gourmelen et al. 1979; Bouchard et al. 1981). In a recent series of ten patients (Gourmelen et al., 1979) the mean basal plasma concentration of 17-hydroxyprogesterone was 4.8 ng/ml compared to 0.4 and 0.3 ng/ml, respectively, in the follicular and luteal phases of the menstrual cycle of normal women. Under ACTH stimulation, plasma 17-hydroxyprogesterone reached a mean value of 50 ng/ml (range: 17–110). In other words, ACTH stimulation multiplied tenfold the baseline values of plasma 17-hydroxyprogesterone.

In conclusion, plasma 17-hydroxyprogesterone levels in partial 21-hydroxylase defect can overlap with the values found in the controls, especially during the luteal phase of the menstrual cycle. Only the dramatic increase of plasma 17-hydroxyprogesterone under ACTH stimulation actually provides evidence of partial 21-hydroxylase deficiency, particularly in cases where the defect is sufficiently mild to prevent the accumulation of precursors under basal conditions.

b) Personal Data

Five women with postpubertal hirsutism due to a partial 21-hydroxylase deficiency were studied. These five cases were selected from an extensive investigation of 250 women who consulted for acquired hirsutism between 1975 and 1979. This small number of patients with 21-hydroxylase defiency gives an idea of the relative rarity of the syndrome. They were compared to three adult women with a complete defect in 21-hydroxylase.

The five women studied were, respectively, 20, 23, 25, 26 and 35 years old. Hirsutism developed after a normal puberty. It was moderate or severe but without male-type muscle increase or clitoromegaly. Clinical history did not show salt-loss syndrome at birth. No family history of salt-loss or hirsutism was noted. Menstrual cycles were ovulatory in the five cases. Two of the patients had had normal pregnancies prior to their first clinical observation. The results of gynaecological examination were normal. No enlarged ovaries were found upon pelvic examination. In summary these patients were often considered as having idiopathic hirsutism.

The three patients with the complete form of 21-hydroxylase deficiency had no salt-loss syndrome but had signs of virilization of the external genitalia at birth and diagnosis had been made during the first years of life. They were studied after interrupting substitutive cortisol treatment for 2 months. At this time they were 25, 30 and 33 years old.

Plasma cortisol, 17-hydroxyprogesterone, testosterone, androstenedione, dehydroisoandrosterone sulphate and urinary 3α-androstanediol were determined by radioimmunoassay (RIA). These determinations were performed during the follicular phase in basal conditions and 1 h after administration of 0.25 mg synthetic ACTH. Blood samples were always collected at 0800 hours. Plasma ACTH was assayed by RIA (Proeschel et al. 1974).

In vitro, skin specimens of pubic origin were obtained from biopsy under local anaesthesia, in four patients with partial 21-hydroxylase deficiency and the three patients with complete defect. Testosterone 5α-reductase activity was measured in a 100 mg sample as previously described (Mauvais-Jarvis et al. 1974: Kuttenn et al. 1977).

The diagnosis of partial 21-hydroxylase deficiency was substantiated by the dramatic increase in 17-hydroxyprogesterone (Fig. 17) after intramuscular injection of 0.25 mg synthetic ACTH, whereas in adult women with 21-hydroxylase deficiency, plasma 17-hydroxyprogesterone was elevated in basal conditions and only slightly increased after ACTH administration. Plasma cortisol levels determined at 0800 hours were lower than normal in both groups, but only slightly in the group with partial 21-hydroxylase deficiency. After ACTH stimulation, plasma cortisol levels remained lower than normal in all patients but with a noticeable increase in patients with partial defect (Fig. 17).

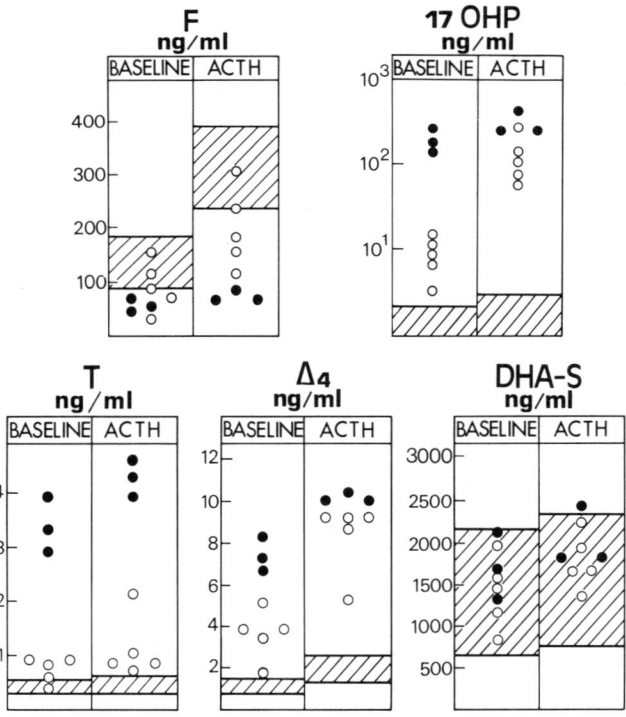

Fig. 17. Plasma levels of cortisol (F), 17–hydroxyprogesterone (17 OHP), testosterone (T), androstenedione (Δ_4) and dehydroisoandrosterone sulphate (DHA-S) before and after IM synthetic ACTH injection, in patients with complete (●) and partial (○) adrenal 21-hydroxylase deficiency. (Normal range for women, mean ± 2 SEM: ▨) Bouchard et al. 1981

Plasma ACTH levels were strongly elevated in patients with the complete 21-hydroxylase defect (260±50 pg/ml), but were normal in patients with partial deficiency (40 pg/ml).

As regards plasma androgens, dehydroisoandrosterone sulphate levels were normal in both groups, in basal conditions as well as after ACTH stimulation. Control values of plasma androstenedione were elevated in both forms of enzyme defect. However, in cases of partial defect, the plasma androstenedione mean value (3.8±1.2 ng/ml) was half that for complete defect (7.2±1.5 ng/ml). After ACTH, the mean plasma androstenedione level was very similar in the two groups of patients (9.2±1.2 and 10.3±1.5 ng/ml, respectively). Plasma testosterone was only slightly elevated in patients with partial enzyme defect and did not increase significantly after ACTH administration. By contrast, in patients with complete defect, basal plasma testosterone was very high (3.5±1.5 ng/ml), but did not increase significantly after ACTH.

Plasma dihydrotestosterone was elevated in patients with the complete enzymatic defect (Fig. 18) but not significantly higher than normal in patients with partial defect, while urinary 3α-androstanediol excretion was clearly elevated in both groups (189±42 and 315±15 μg/24 h, respectively).

In vitro (Fig. 18), testosterone 5α-reductase activity was found normal or subnormal in the four studied cases with partial defect, whereas the range for 5α-reductase activity was always higher than normal in the three patients with complete defect.

When the five patients studied were compared to others with complete 21-hydroxylase defect, it appeared obvious that the enzymatic block was only partial. In these five patients, in basal conditions plasma 17-hydroxyprogesterone was only slightly higher than normal, but showed a dramatic increase after ACTH administration. By contrast, in patients with complete enzymatic defect, 17-hydroxyprogesterone was considerably high in basal conditions and showed no increase after ACTH administration.

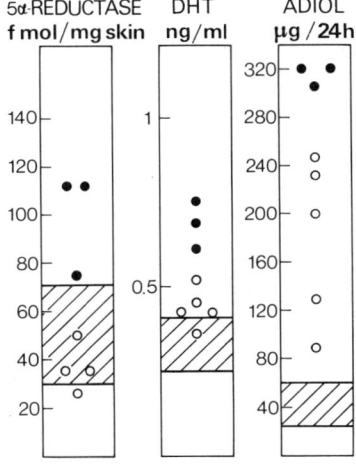

Fig. 18. Parameters of target organ "utilization" of androgens: skin 5α-reductase activity, plasma dihydrotestosterone (*DHT*) and urinary 3α-androstanediol excretion (*Adiol*) in patients with complete (●) and partial (○) adrenal 21-hydroxylase deficiency. (Normal range for women, mean ±2 SEM: ▨) Bouchard et al., 1981

c) Interpretation of Results

These observations correlate with the values of plasma ACTH obtained in the two groups of patients. Plasma ACTH is markedly high in the complete form of 21-hydroxylase defect, whereas the normal values of plasma ACTH observed in patients with acquired virilization indicate that, at least in basal conditions, without any stress or physical or psychological stimulation of ACTH production, the merely partial defect in 17-hydroxylase permits sufficient cortisol production to exert normal, negative feedback on ACTH production (Pham-Huu-Trung et al. 1979).

Hirsutism in patients with partial defect in 21-hydroxylase seems to be induced by the increase of androstenedione production. The deficiency in 21-hydroxylase leads to an increase in 17-hydroxyprogesterone biosynthesis. 17-Hydroxyprogesterone is metabolized through alternate pathways: to either pregnanetriol (Fukushima et al. 1961) or androstenedione (Rivarola et al. 1967a). In patients with partial defect, most of the plasma testosterone originates from conversion of androstenedione. However, in patients with complete defect one cannot eliminate a direct secretion of testosterone by adrenals, as noted by other authors (Burger et al. 1964).

5α-Reductase activity differs according to the type of 21-hydroxylase deficiency. In the complete form it is elevated. This may be due to the increased secretion of testosterone by the adrenals which may stimulate 5α-reductase activity in the skin, as observed in men at puberty (Mauvais-Jarvis 1977). In patients with partial defect, 5α-reductase activity is within the normal range for normal women. It is far lower than in idiopathic hirsutism. These data suggest that in patients with partial 21-hydroxylase deficiency the major factor which seems to be responsible for virilization is the elevated production of androstenedione. By contrast, there is no increased "utilization" of androgens by the skin as is observed in idiopathic hirsutism (see Sect. K.III.3b).

6. Identification of the Heterozygous State

Congenital adrenal hyperplasia due to 21-hydroxylase deficiency is inherited as an autosomal recessive trait (Childs et al. 1956; Prader et al. 1962), the heterozygous individuals being clinically indistinguishable from normal subjects (Knorr et al. 1977). The accurate detection of heterozygotes is of more than theoretical interest because of the implications of genetic considerations. The problem is not as crucial in the delayed onset forms as in the precocious forms. Nevertheless, as long as the exact relationship between the two disorders has not been clearly established, and considering the frequency of heterozygotes in the general population (1:40), it would seem useful to favour such a prospective study.

Early attempts to identify the heterozygous state by measurement of urinary 17-ketosteroids and pregnanetriol after ACTH stimulation were only partially successful (Childs et al. 1956; Cleveland et al. 1962; Hall et al. 1970). More recently, the acute response of plasma 17-hydroxyprogesterone to ACTH administration was found to be significantly greater in heterozygotes than in unaffected homozygotes (Lee and Gareis 1975; Knorr et al. 1975; Gutai et al. 1977; Krensky et al. 1977). In addition, after ACTH, higher levels of plasma 17-hydroxyprogesterone were observed in heterozygous individuals than in controls, indicating a partial defect in 21-hydroxylase (Rosenwaks et al. 1979). However, because there was considerable overlapping between normal and carrier values, ACTH stimulation is not reliable for diagnosis of heterozygote carriers in all instances (Lee and Gareis 1975).

7. Genetic Linkage Between 21-Hydroxylase Deficiency and the HLA Blood Group System

The gene for congenital adrenal hyperplasia due to 21-hydroxylase deficiency is located on chromosome 6, close to the HLA-B locus (Dupont et al. 1977). HLA typing did not show a difference in the HLA antigens among salt-losing and non-salt-losing patients. Both forms are in very close genetic linkage with HLA-B. The genes for the 21-hydroxylase enzymes of the mineralocorticoid and glucocorticoid pathways are located close to the locus for the HLA-B determinants.

The heterogeneity described in the phenotypic expression of the 21-hydroxylase deficiency may be caused by environmental factors and/or genes not linked to the HLA complex, more or less compensating for this hormonal disorder. Another explanation would be to assume that the 21-hydroxylase deficiency is coded not only by one gene, but rather by two or more genes (Bartter et al. 1968) closely linked and located within the HLA complex. Since 21-hydroxylase acts within different biosynthetic pathways, producing either cortisol or aldosterone, one might argue that in each of these pathways, 21-hydroxylases with different substrate specificities are involved. Assuming that these different 21-hydroxylases are under the genetic control of different but closely linked genes and that for each of these genes defective variants do exist, the different phenotypes of congenital adrenal hyperplasia would be the result of varying combinations of normal and defective 21-hydroxylase genes in either a homozygous or heterozygous state.

There is a lack of association between 21-hydroxylase deficiency gene and any of the known HLA-A, HLA-B and HLA-C antigens. This lack demonstrates a random association between alleles of HLA loci and the 21-hydroxylase locus, in spite of the close genetic linkage.

These findings support the concept that 21-hydroxylase deficiency occurs as a result of multiple unrelated mutations and that such mutation is relatively common.

As a result of linkage to the HLA group, it is possible to accurately predict heterozygosity of the gene for 21-hydroxylase deficiency in siblings of affected parents. The consideration of HLA typing and biological testing is the most precise tool for recognizing 21-hydroxylase deficiency carriers in families with authenticated disease.

To date, most studies on genetic linkage to the HLA system have only concerned the complete defect in 21-hydroxylase. Studies on HLA in partial defect (delayed onset congenital adrenal hyperplasia) remain scarce and controversial (New et al. 1979). In recent studies not yet published (Boue et al., Dupont et al.) concerning 10 families, a linkage with the HLA system contrary to that observed by New et al. (1979) was found. Additional data are thus required to determine whether precocious and delayed onset forms of 21-hydroxylase deficiency are of identical origin.

8. Treatment

From a pathological point of view, the treatment of congenital adrenal hyperplasia is based upon the correction of the cortisol biosynthesis deficiency.

a) Corticosteroid Replacement

Two types of therapy are used: natural compounds, e. g. cortisol and cortisone, or long-acting synthetic corticosteroids such as dexamethasone (Riddick and Hammond 1975a). The doses usually proposed are based on corresponding biological effects. Most authors are far from unanimous concerning the appropriate therapy, particularly in the case of the partial defect in 21-hydroxylase. However, it seems logical to propose to women after puberty a treatment without side effects, such as cortisol (hydrocortisone) in doses of 20–30 mg/day. The dramatic response of plasma steroids to a single dose of hydrocortisone indicates that the hypothalamic pituitary adrenal axis of patients with 21-hydroxylase deficiency is highly sensitive to cortisol. However, this effect may be short lived (Brook et al. 1974; Lippe et al. 1974).

In fact, adequate therapy in patients with 21-hydroxylase deficiency constantly comes up against two obstacles: (1) the persistence of a nycthemeral cycle of ACTH secretion, with a peak after midnight (Fukushima et al. 1975); and (2) the increase in the need of cortisol and in turn the increase in ACTH secretion in case of stress. It is therefore difficult to control efficiently the androgen overproduction which directly depends on the ACTH production. An effort must thus be made to use minimal doses of hydrocortisone, to avoid side effects due to overdosage, and to give the larger fraction of the cortisol therapy in the late evening, to suppress the nocturnal surge of ACTH. However, cortisone therapy in parallel with variable daily needs has, of course, not yet been monitored.

The biological control of treatment is difficult and controversial. *Plasma 17-hydroxyprogesterone* determinations under treatment, alone or associated with ACTH stimulation, have been proposed (Pham-Huu-Trung et al. 1978) as an index of therapeutic adequacy. However, many patients with good control have plasma 17-hydroxyprogesterone levels greater than the maximal values shown in normal subjects (Lippe et al. 1974). Indeed, patients suffering 21-hydroxylase deficiency have high plasma 17-hydroxyprogesterone concentration, because their steroidogenesis is blocked at this stage. Normalizing 17-hydroxyprogesterone production therefore implies running a risk of suppressing steroidogenesis to a subnormal rate by using supraphysiological cortisol doses.

Testosterone determination is not a good index of treatment adequacy since this androgen mainly originates from the conversion of androstenedione. The determination of plasma *androstenedione* seems the better index for adrenal suppression and control of hirsutism, since androstenedione is the main androgen secreted in this disease (Horton and Frasier 1967; Rivarola et al. 1967a; Gandy and Peterson 1968; Korth-Schutz et al. 1978).

b) Other Treatments

Due to the difficulty in providing adequate androgen suppression, hirsutism remains hard to control with mere cortisol therapy. It therefore appears that inhibition of peripheral androgen action should be considered. Certain authors have tried oestrogen-progestagen combinations (Brooks et al. 1960; Riddick and

Hammond 1975 a), but such combinations intensify the side effects of cortisone treatment without any real improvement in the development of hirsutism. Conventional oestrogen-progestagen association currently tends to be replaced by combinations using true antiandrogens, particularly *cyproterone acetate*. In addition to the antigonadotropic effect which inhibits ovarian androgen secretion, and its peripheral antiandrogenic effect, cyproterone acetate seems to have an inhibitory action on adrenal biosythesis (Girard et al. 1978; Panesar and Stitch 1976). Thus, this therapeutic agent may be of help in allowing a decrease in suppressive doses of cortisone.

II. Congenital Adrenal Hyperplasia Due to 11β-Hydroxylase Deficiency

Adrenogenital syndrome due to 11β-hydroxylase deficiency was first described by Eberlein and Bongiovanni (1955). It is rarer than 21-hydroxylase deficiency, and its clinical picture consists of virilization associated with hypertension.

1. Pathophysiology

The defect in 11β-hydroxylase results in deficient cortisol secretion and leads to hypersecretion of ACTH. ACTH is responsible for cortical adrenal hyperplasia and an excessive production of cortisol precursors, such as 11-deoxycortisol (compound S), the steroid immediately preceding the enzymatic defect (see Table 8). On the biosynthetic pathway of cortisol, there is also an excessive synthesis of 17-hydroxyprogesterone which therefore bypasses the cortisol biosynthetic pathway and leads to an excess of androgen production — essentially androstenedione and, to a lesser extent, testosterone. The 11β-hydroxylase deficiency also concerns the biosynthesis of aldosterone, resulting in an excessive production of 11-deoxycorticosterone, the steroid immediately preceding the enzymatic defect. The abnormal production of 11-deoxycorticosterone is responsible for hypertension. Plasma aldosterone levels, which are low in untreated patients, surprisingly increase when cortisol therapy is undertaken (New and Seaman 1970). As in 21-hydroxylase deficiency, the 11β-hydroxylase defect appears more pronounced in the cortisol rather than the aldosterone biosynthetic pathway. Is it due to different affinities of the enzyme for different substrates (17-hydroxylated or not deoxycorticosterone)? Or is it simply due to the normal disproportion between the respective need and production of cortisol and aldosterone (the former being 150 times greater than the latter)?

For several authors, the adrenal gland appears to behave as two glands: the fasciculata and the glomerulosa (New and Seaman 1970; West et al. 1979; Levine et al. 1980). The glomerulosa regulated by the renin-angiotensin system produces aldosterone. This production is suppressed when the fasciculata secretes an excess of 11-deoxycorticosterone which in turn decreases the renin secretion. The 11β-hydroxylase deficiency might occur mainly in the fasciculata zone which is regulated by ACTH. When ACTH is suppressed by dexamethasone, the fasciculata stops secreting 11-deoxycorticosterone, thus permitting the zona glomerulosa to synthesize aldosterone under the control of the derepressed renin. This would support two separate 11β-hydroxylase enzymatic systems.

2. Clinical Features

This form of congenital adrenal hyperplasia is rare. As with 21-hydroxylase deficiency, it may present different clinical expressions from the most severe syndrome, with female pseudohermaphroditism at birth and salt-loss, to the mildest form with simple delayed onset hirsutism (Brooks et al. 1960; Gabrilove et al. 1965; Schaison and Gilbert-Dreyfus 1974; Newmark et al. 1977). In the delayed onset form of this syndrome patients are generally of short stature, they have severe hirsutism with only slight virilization of the external genitalia and menstrual disorders are observed. The presence of an elevated blood pressure is also very suggestive of the diagnosis (Zachman and Prader 1980). However, the clinical picture may be less obvious when the patients shows an isolated hirsutism with ovulatory cycle and no hypertension.

3. Hormonal Characteristics

Urinary 17-ketosteroid analysis is not helpful for diagnosis of this form of congenital adrenal hyperplasia. However, the simultaneous increase in urinary 17-ketosteroids and 17-hydroxycorticosteroids is more significant. This last increase is due to the elevated urinary excretion of tetrahydro -S (Green et al. 1960). A suppressive test using dexamethasone leads to the decrease of both urinary 17-ketosteroids and 17-hydroxycorticosteroids (Liddle 1960). This test is supposed to distinguish suppressible from non-suppressible oversecretions, such as virilizing tumours or Cushing's disease.

It is therefore more accurate to measure plasma cortisol and its precursors before and after ACTH (Pham-Huu-Trung et al. 1973; Gourmelen et al. 1979). If, after ACTH, plasma cortisol increase is inadequate, other plasma assays may then be performed, in particular, 11-deoxycortisol (compound S) and 17-hydroxyprogesterone. These plasma determinations thus permit an assured diagnosis.

4. Genetic Transmission

11β-Hydroxylase deficiency is a recessive transmitted disorder. HLA typing in families with 11β-hydroxylase has revealed the absence of linkage to the HLA system (Brautbar et al. 1979).

5. Treatment

Cortisol replacement suppresses the abnormal ACTH overproduction and then corrects the elevated secretion of both androgens and desoxycorticosterone. This treatment rapidly corrects the hypertension (Wilkins et al. 1952). Its effect on hirsutism is not so marked as in 21-hydroxylase deficiency.

III. Virilizing Adrenal Tumours

First included in the adrenogenital syndrome described by Apert (1910) and Gallais (1912), virilizing adrenal tumours were then individualized. They have certain practically constant characteristics, in particular a rapid onset virilization syndrome due to an overproduction of weak androgens, but in enormous quantities; this secretion is neither stimulated by ACTH nor suppressed by dexamethasone.

1. Pathology

This has been studied by various authors (Huvos et al. 1970; Harrison et al. 1973).

a) Macroscopy

Macroscopically, the tumour is round shaped or sometimes uneven and may weigh a few hundred grams. When sectioned, the texture is homogenous and yellow coloured or, in other cases, heterogeneous and brittle, with haemorrhagic and necrotic zones. The controlateral adrenal gland is usually atrophic. Some rare possibilities exist e. g. bilateral localization and ectopic tumour (Birke et al. 1958) adjacent to a polyadenomatous adrenal gland. The tumoral derivation from previous congenital hyperplasia has been discussed (Hamvi et al. 1957; Dluly et al. 1971).

b) Histology

Histologically, these tumours originate from the fascicula-reticula zone. There are two cytologic types: (1) *orthoplasic* tumours in which the structure is adenomorphic and homogeneous; the nucleus is monomorphic, and mitoses are absent; and (2) *anaplasic* tumours, in which the structure is anarchic with zones of oedema, necrosis and haemorrhage. The nuclei are large with numerous mitoses.

c) Malignant Criteria

The difficulty in predicting the clinical behaviour of virilizing adrenal tumours on the basis of their histologic appearance is well documented (Symington 1963).

Enlarged vesicular nuclei, mitotic activity, extensive areas of necrosis and haemorrhage and capsular and venous invasion are more prominent in the malignant tumours. Frequently, however, malignant cortical tumours may display remarkable uniformity with little pleomorphism or mitotic activity. Thus, many tumours thought to be benign upon surgery and histological examination, have been followed by recurrence and late metastases. That is why any virilizing adrenal tumour must be considered, to various degrees, as having a potential for malignancy!

2. Steroid Production

Adrenal carcinomas associated with excessive production of glucocorticoids, androgens and oestrogens and with the clinical manifestations of Cushing's syndrome, hyperaldosteronism, virilization or feminization, have been reported.

In fact, virilizing adrenal tumours generally show two different secretory profiles: (1) isolated virilization exclusively due to an androgen overproduction and (2) virilization associated with symptoms of Cushing's syndrome reflecting a mixed oversecretion of androgens and glucocorticoids (Hutter and Kayhoe, 1966a). Due to their exceptional androgen overproduction, far greater than in physiological conditions, adrenal tumours have fundamentally contributed to the knowledge of adrenal steroidogenesis. Indeed, biosynthetic pathways are the same in adrenal tumours as in normal adrenals, but some are amplified and steroids that are usually only precursors for physiological hormonal secretion can themselves become secretory products (Baulieu et al. 1967).

Normal adrenal androgen secretion consists mainly of weak androgens, which are produced through two different pathways. The first (Δ_5 pathway) originates from pregnenolone which is transformed into 17-hydroxypregnenolone and then into dehydroisoandrosterone (particularly in its sulphate form) and into androstenediol. The second pathway (Δ_4 pathway) originates from progesterone which is transformed into 17-hydroxyprogesterone and then into androstenedione and 11 β-hydroxyandrostenedione. Testosterone is normally secreted weakly, if at all, by the adrenals.

a) Dehydroisoandrosterone

The enormous production of dehydroisoandrosterone, particularly of dehydroisoandrosterone sulphate, has been demonstrated by incubation techniques and assays in efferent venous blood from adrenal tumours (Baulieu et al. 1967; Saez et al. 1967; Mahesh et al. 1968). These experiments have demonstrated that in adrenal tumours the Δ_5-androgen biosynthetic pathway is generally predominant. According to Dorfman et al. (1963) it would be due to a relative insufficiency of the 3β-ol, dehydrogenase enzyme, the Δ_5/Δ_4 pathway ratio depending on this enzymatic activity. This weak enzymatic activity could also explain the overproduction of dehydroisoandrosterone. Indeed, dehydroisoandrosterone sulphate is synthesized in enormous quantities: up to 100 times the normal values. This explains how adrenal sulphatase was first observed in tumoral adrenal tissue.

b) Other Androgens

Androstenedione and 11β-hydroxyandrostenedione have been found to be produced in excess by adrenal tumours. However, since these steroids are produced along the Δ_4 pathway, their overproduction remains far from dehydroisoandrosterone overproduction. *Testosterone* synthesis has been demonstrated in steroid extractions from adrenal tumours (Anliker et al. 1956) and assays in adrenal venous blood (Saez et al. 1967; Mahesh et al. 1968).

3. Clinical Aspects of Virilizing Adrenal Tumours

Carcinomas of the adrenal cortex are uncommon tumours. Two-thirds of patients with this disease are women, perhaps because the endocrine syndrome helps earlier diagnosis (Lipsett et al. 1963).

a) Adult Females

In adult females, these tumours usually occur between 30 and 40 years of age; however, tumours occurring after menopause are not exceptional (Hutter and Kayhoe 1966 a).

In most patients, hirsutism is the first clinical symptom. It is of dramatically rapid and generalized onset. The skin becomes thick, and acne and seborrhoea extensively develop, accompanied by progressive alopecia. Hirsutism is associated with other marked symptoms of virilization; clitoral hypertrophy is frequently observed, and there is often hypertrophy of the labia majora which become hyperpigmented. Muscular hypertrophy with loss of the characteristic female fat deposits gives the body a masculine appearance. The voice also progressively deepens. Apart from the symptoms of virilization there are also some signs of defeminization. Menstrual disorders are constant; oligomenorrhoea is first observed quickly followed by complete amenorrhoea. Atrophy of the breasts is also generally observed.

b) Prepubertal Females

In prebubertal females, a rapid statural growth is observed in addition to the development of hirsutism and the enlargement of the clitoris. A marked advance in bone maturation may be noted, which results in rapid closure of the epiphysis, and the patient will not achieve full growth. In addition, no breast development occurs at puberty and the menses do not appear. Only on exceptional occasions can the clinical examination of the lumbar fossa and hypochondriac regions reveal the presence of an adrenal tumour.

4. Hormonal Findings

a) Urinary Steroids

Virilizing adrenal tumours are probably the only cause of hirsutism for which the determination of urinary 17-ketosteroids remains helpful for diagnosis. Urinary 17-ketosteroids are, indeed, dramatically elevated. Levels of up to 200 mg/24 h are not exceptional (Lipsett et al. 1963; Hutter and Kayhoe 1966 a). This increase is essentially due to the overproduction of dehydroisoandrosterone sulphate by the tumour (Baulieu 1962; Lipsett et al., 1963; Hutter and Kayhoe 1966 a; Nogeire et al. 1977). Androsterone, aetiocholanolone and 11β-hydroxyandrosterone also contribute to the increase of 17-ketosteroids, but never in the same proportion as dehydroisoandrosterone. Urinary testosterone glucuronide has also been found to be elevated (Futterweit et al. 1964), as well as urinary androstane -3β, 17β-diol. An increase in urinary excretion of some metabolites of androgen precursors has also been observed in particular, pregnanediol and pregnanetriol (Kapler et al. 1948; Lipsett and Wilson 1962). Reflecting the more or less associated excess of glucocorticoid biosynthesis, urinary 17-hydroxycorticosteroid levels vary from normal to high, reaching 40–100 mg/24 h.

b) Plasma Steroids

The steroid recovered in the greatest amount in the plasma of patients with virilizing adrenal tumours is indeed dehydroisoandrosterone, particularly in its sulphate form (Baulieu 1962; Saez et al. 1967; Nogeire et al. 1977). Plasma androstenedione, and to a lesser extent, plasma testosterone levels are elevated but variable: from 2–20 times the values observed in normal women (Saez et al. 1967; Bardin et al. 1968).

c) Dynamic Tests

Adrenal tumours are usually autonomous and do not react to either stimulating or suppressive dynamic tests. The administration of ACTH has generally no effect on plasma or urinary steroid levels. However, several authors have reported some cases of adrenal tumours responding to ACTH (Mahesh et al. 1968). Suppressive tests using dexamethasone are generally ineffective. Here again some authors have noted a significant suppression of hormonal levels in some cases (Korth-Schutz et al. 1977).

In addition, stimulation with HCG has been observed as positive in some cases of adrenal tumours (Werk et al. 1973; Givens et al. 1974; Blichert-Toft et al. 1975), and it can therefore be concluded that dynamic tests are not reliable for the diagnosis of adrenal tumours or for all virilizing syndromes.

5. Physical Methods for Diagnosis of Virilizing Adrenal Tumours

In most cases, the diagnosis of virilizing adrenal tumours is based on clinical features, i.e. the rapid development of a major hirsutism accompanied by other signs of virilization. The hormonal findings are generally characteristic, in particular the increase of urinary 17-ketosteroids and plasma dehydroisoandrosterone sulphate which are not suppressed by dexamethasone. In some cases, however the clinical and biological features may not be so clear cut particularly when the androgen secretion consists essentially of testosterone and when dexamethasone has an unexpected suppressive effect (Korth-Schutz et al. 1977). In such cases, the visualization of the tumour by physical methods becomes necessary.

It is not exceptional for the tumour to be visible in a simple X-ray examination such as a standard abdominal examination, *uronephrogram* with tomography, which shows a rounded suprarenal mass weighing the kidney outwards and downwards. Otherwise, *echography* (Birnholz 1973) and/or *scanning* can help diagnosis by defining size, extent and anatomic site of the tumour. *Scintigraphy* of the adrenals using 131-I-iodo-cholesterol can provide a visual display of structure and function of the adrenal tumour (Seabold and Schteingart 1975; Barbarino et al. 1976; Sarkar et al. 1977).

These various examinations are particularly well tolerated and sufficiently reliable to lessen the need for *arteriography and phlebography*. The latter two, especially when Cushing's syndrome is associated with virilization, indeed present great vascular risks: haemorrhage and thrombo-embolism, due to the extreme fragility of the vessels of these patients. Nevertheless, when all the physical explorations do not provide conclusive results, *venous catheterization* can be performed percutaneously via the femoral vein. Catheters are selectively threaded into adrenal veins on both sides for blood sampling. Testosterone, androstenedione, dehydroisoandrosterone sulphate, oestradiol and cortisol are assayed in these samples, and their concentrations are compared to peripheral concentrations. According to Kirschner et al. (1976c), the mean adrenal effluent level for testosterone is normally 2.6 times that of peripheral blood. The gradient for androstenedione is 6.0; for dehydroisoandrosterone, 100; and for cortisol, 23.

During venous catheterization, the blood sampling can be done in association with venography (Gabrilove et al. 1976). After the blood sample has been obtained, radiocontrast material is injected for visualization of the expected adrenal tumour.

6. Treatment

The treatment of virilizing adrenal tumours is both surgical and medical.

a) Surgical

This should be performed whenever the tumour appears well circumscribed, even if pulmonary metastases exist, since metastases may disappear under chemotherapy. Patients successfully operated on experienced a marked decrease in hirsutism, a return of the menses, but only a slow and often incomplete regression of other symptoms of virilization.

b) Chemotherapy

Mitotane (ortho-para'-dichloro-diphenyl-dichloromethane, OP'DDD) has a dual action: it inhibits adrenal steroid biosynthesis (Touitou et al. 1977, 1978) and it has an antimitotic effect and induces necrosis and regression of adrenal secretory carcinomas (Bergenstal et al. 1960; Hutter and Kayhoe 1966b; Lubitz et al. 1973; Becker and Schumacher 1975; Bricaire and Luton 1977). OP'DDD is used at a dose of 12 g/day, per os. This treatment is indicated when metastases exist. In addition, OP'DDD might be used systematically after surgery, even in the absence of metastases, considering the potential malignant evolution of virilizing adrenal tumours. OP'DDD has considerably increased patient survival in the two-thirds of patients who proved "responders" to this treatment (Hutter and Kayhoe 1966b; Lubitz et al. 1973; Bricaire and Luton 1977).

The evolution of the tumour, or of its metastases, can be followed through urinary 17-ketosteroid excretion or even better with plasma androgen determination. In patients showing tumour recurrence or metastases occurrence, an increase in androgen levels is generally observed. After 4 weeks of treatment with OP'DDD, a decrease in these levels is only observed in "responders".

c) Benign Tumours

When most arguments (macroscopical and histological) support benignity of the tumour and if surgical treatment has been definite, no additional treatment is necessary. Indeed in most cases, one may observe, in a relatively short time, a complete disappearance of hirsutism; this is contrary to that observed in other cases of non-tumoral hirsutism.

J. Hirsutism of Ovarian Origin

I. Polycystic Ovarian Syndrome

Polycystic ovarian syndrome was first described by Stein and Leventhal (1935) as an anovulatory syndrome with menstrual cycle disorders, sterility, virilization and increased size of the ovaries. These clinical and anatomical features were quickly found to be an insufficient description, and many authors tried to elucidate the physiopathology of this syndrome, the main question being: Is this syndrome of hypothalamopituitary or ovarian origin? Methodological progress in hormonology, especially radioimmunoassays and dynamic stimulation tests, now allows a better understanding of the mechanism, and even though these tests do not assure the causal lesion, they provide a good definition of the characteristic features of this syndrome at both the hypothalamopituitary and ovarian levels.

1. Theory of "Hypothalamic Masculinization"

Neonatal hypothalamic virilization in the female rat receiving high androgen doses at birth, with ensuing destruction of the anterior cyclic part of the hypothalamic center, was long considered a good physiopathological model (Barraclough et al. 1961). Androgen administration in the neonatal period in rats induces a permanent oestrus and polycystic ovaries.

In fact, this model is not applicable to primates. Yamaji et al. (1971), studying the neuroendocrinological control of ovulation in rhesus monkeys, have shown that the tonic pituitary secretion of FSH and LH is controlled by an oestradiol-negative feedback, but it is disrupted every 28 days by an LH surge and, to a lesser extent, FSH, responding to the plasma oestradiol peak with, at that time, a positive feedback effect. Contrary to that observed in the rat, the surgical deafferentation of the basal medial hypothalamus does not alter the hypothalamic tonic secretion and does not suppress the estrogen-induced LH surge.

Non-definitive hypothalamic virilization has been observed in the human species. Kulin and Reiter (1976) succeeded in inducing an LH surge in male as well as female adults after several days of highly dosed oestrogen treatment.

2. Two Types of Polycystic Ovaries

Yen et al. (1970a) described a special gonadotropin secretion in 16 cases of polycystic ovaries, which was characterized by a constantly elevated plasma LH level with no cyclic surge, contrasting with a normal or low plasma FSH level. Gambrell et al. (1973) only found such data in some patients: in 26 patients with polycystic ovaries, FSH plasma levels were constantly low, but LH was high, normal or low. Givens et al. (1976c) showed that there are two groups of patients with polycystic ovaries: one with high plasma LH levels and the other with normal LH secretion. HCG stimulation provokes plasma testosterone and Δ_4-androstenedione increase, only in the normal LH group. By contrast, in high plasma LH cases, no testosterone or androstenedione increase was observed after HCG stimulation, the ovarian stroma secretion being already stimulated by endogenous LH.

Berger et al. (1975) confirmed the existence of two polycystic ovary groups, with regards to basal plasma LH and FSH levels. In the type I polycystic ovary, LH was high and FSH normal. These patients had more marked amenorrhoea or oligomenorrhoea. The ovaries were enlarged ($\times 2$ or $\times 4$); anatomopathological examination revealed a stromal hyperplasia and a thick cortex under which lay microcystic primary follicles. In the type II polycystic ovary, plasma LH was high but less so than in group I and with minor pulses; FSH was constantly low. The ovaries were not as enlarged as in the first group; they also had stromal hyperplasia and follicular cysts.

Group I is very close to the syndrome described by Stein and Leventhal. Group II is more heterogeneous and the polycystic ovaries very often appear secondary to mechanical, infectious, psychological or endocrinological diseases, especially of adrenal origin.

3. LH-RH Test in the Polycystic Ovarian Syndrome

Rebar et al. (1976) also found two types of gonadotropic secretion in polycystic ovaries: (1) high plasma LH and normal or low plasma FSH, and (2) slightly elevated plasma LH and low plasma FSH. The amplitude of LH secretory pulses is very high in type I, but in addition the frequency of these pulses is higher. The LH-RH stimulation induces a dramatic increase in LH in type I polycystic ovaries, whereas the response is subnormal in type II cases. Moreover, iterative injections of small doses of LH-RH (10 µg/2 h) immediately stimulate major LH secretion, expressing an increased pituitary sensitivity to LH-RH (Fig. 19). Rebar et al. (1976) emphasize the parallel between the response to LH-RH and plasma oestradiol plus oestrone levels.

4. Clomiphene Test

This test explores the hypothalamic secretory capacity. It indirectly stimulates endogenous LH-RH secretion: clomiphene citrate is a competitive inhibitor of oestradiol-binding hypothalamus receptors. At a 100 mg/day dose for 5 days, it temporarily blocks oestradiol binding if plasma oestradiol level is sufficient (See Fig. 20). It thus momentarily inhibits the negative feedback due to ovarian tonic oestradiol secretion. (Yen et al. 1970b)

As early as 1969, Mauvais-Jarvis et al. observed an increase in LH and even FSH during the clomiphene test, in patients with the polycystic ovary syndrome. This gonadotropic increase permits a follicular maturation otherwise impossible due to the low FSH levels. Plasma oestradiol increases up to preovulatory levels. The subsequent LH peak induces ovulation, and progesterone secretion and thermal plateau ensue. Yen et al. (1970a, 1976) confirmed positiveness of this test in the polycystic ovary syndrome, and concluded that the hypothalamic positive feedback due to oestradiol is maintained. This test is also used in treatment for sterility: using

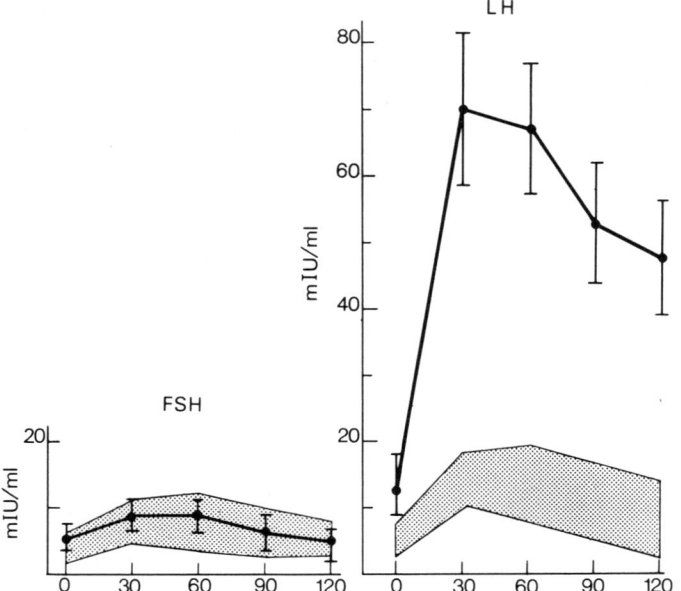

Fig. 19. FSH and LH release in response to 100 µg of LH-RH in 12 women with polycystic ovaries syndrome compared to 10 normal women explored during early luteal phase of cycle (mean ± SEM). *PCO*, polycystic ovary. Mauvais-Jarvis et al. 1978

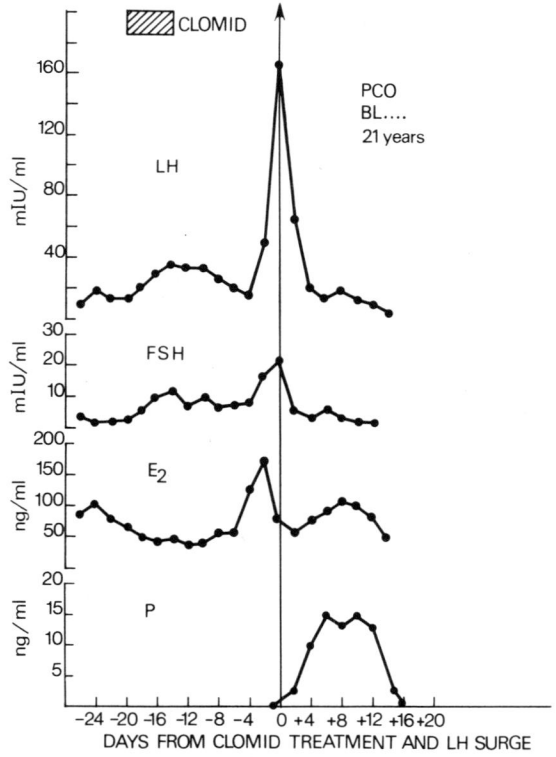

Fig. 20. Effect on plasma FSH, LH, oestradiol (E_2) and progesterone (P) of a daily administration of 100 mg clomiphene for 5 days in a case of polycystic ovarian syndrome (*PCO*). Mauvais-Jarvis et al. 1978

it, Mauvais-Jarvis et al. (1978) induced ten pregnancies in 15 patients with polycystic ovaries.

5. Oestradiol Test

The administration of sufficient oestradiol doses helps evaluate the negative feedback of this steroid. Rebar et al. (1976) perfused oestradiol, 50 pg/h for 4 h and plasma oestradiol concentrations increased up to 300–800 pg/ml. In all the patients, LH decreased markedly and returned to normal only after the end of the perfusion. These results suggest that negative feedback is intact in this affection.

6. Androgen Overproduction in Polycystic Ovarian Syndrome (Fig. 21)

As early as 1967, Bardin and Lipsett showed that in polycystic ovaries there is an ovarian overproduction of testosterone and especially androstenedione, the main ovary-produced androgen, as well as an increase in testosterone metabolic clearance that is between the rate for normal women (700 1/24 h) and normal men (1250 1/24 h). In women with polycystic ovaries, the percentage of testosterone derived from androstenedione (26%) is less than in normal women (50%). During the same period, Rivarola et al. (1967 b) catheterized ovarian veins and found more than normal amounts of testosterone and androstenedione coming from polycystic ovaries. Kirschner et al. (1976 a) observed that the androstenedione concentration was 20 times higher in blood samples taken from ovarian veins than in those taken from peripheral ones. On the other hand, in these patients dehydroisoandrosterone provides only 6% of plasma androstenedione and 0.6% of testosterone. Women suffering from polycystic ovaries therefore present a consistent hormonal profile, i.e. high plasma androstenedione which can reach twice normal values (between 3 and 5 ng/ml) (Southren et al. 1969 b; Mahoudeau et al. 1971; Kuttenn et al. 1977). Such a rise in androstenedione production may alone explain the moderate increase in testosterone production due to hepatic and extrahepatic metabolism; however, a

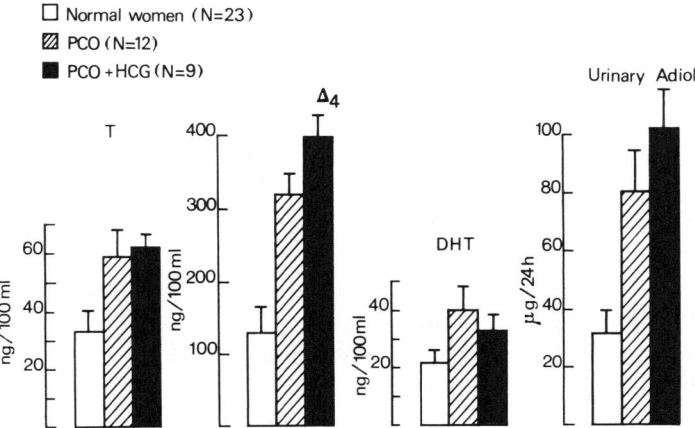

Fig. 21. Plasma testosterone (T), androstenedione (Δ_4), dihydrotestosterone (DHT) and urinary 3α-androstanediol (*Adiol*) in women with polycystic ovary values before (▨) and after (■) 15 000 IU HCG, compared with normal women (□). *PCO*, polycystic ovary; *N*, number. Mauvais-Jarvis et al. 1978

moderate testosterone oversecretion by the ovary itself is probable (Kirschner et al. 1976 a). This increase in plasma testosterone is responsible for a decrease in TeBG capacity (Southren et al. 1968) and consequently for an increase in the plasma free testosterone and in its metabolic clearance rate (Vermeulen et al., 1969).

Concerning androgen sensitivity in the skin, hirsute women with polycystic ovaries have an increased 5α-reductase activity (Kuttenn and Mauvais-Jarvis, 1975; Mauvais-Jarvis et al. 1976 a, b; Kuttenn et al. 1977). The skin can therefore utilize all available androgen substrates: free testosterone and above all androstenedione which is not bound to TeBG but passively diffuses into the skin and may thus be locally converted to testosterone and dihydrotestosterone by increased local 5α-reductase activity (Gomez and Hsia 1968, Kuttenn et al. 1977). This results in an excess of urinary 3α-androstanediol excretion (Mauvais-Jarvis et al. 1974). Actually, 3α-androstanediol may be considered a terminal metabolite of both testosterone and androstenedione (Mahoudeau et al. 1971; Kuttenn et al. 1977). In women with polycystic ovaries, urinary 3α-androstanediol excretion is close to male levels (Mauvais-Jarvis et al. 1973; Kuttenn et al. 1977). This increased urinary excretion reflects, on the one hand, androstenedione overproduction by the ovary, and on the other hand, the excess conversion by skin of androstenedione into testosterone and then into dihydrotestosterone and 3α-androstanediol.

It should also be noted that certain assays such as urinary 17-ketosteroids and other tests such as dexamethasone-HCG, are of little help in diagnosing the origin of hirsutism. 17-Ketosteroids are terminal metabolites from both ovarian and adrenal biosynthesis. The major part derives from androgens but another part does come from glucocorticoids (11-keto or 11-hydroxy-glucocorticoids).

The dexamethasone-HCG stimulation-suppression test which is supposed to discriminate between ovarian and adrenal androgen overproduction, also seems to lack precision: (1) dexamethasone not only suppresses adrenal biosynthesis, but also ovarian biosynthesis; (2) adrenal suppression is most efficient on glucocorticoids, but incomplete on androgens after only 6 days of dexamethasone administration; and (3) ovarian dystrophy which should be revealed by this test, can be one of the two types: type I, with high LH and no androgen response to HCG stimulation, or type II with less elevated LH and positive response to HCG. It is therefore obvious that the lack of specificity of this test makes it inaccurate.

7. Pathophysiology of Polycystic Ovarian Syndrome

Based on the various studies in the last 10 years, the following observations can be made:

In the complete form of the syndrome, plasma LH is high, with higher and more frequent pulses than normal.

This LH level increases dramatically when stimulated by exogenous LH-RH and the response to iterative LH-RH stimulation leads us to believe that there is an increased pituitary sensitivity to LH-RH rather than an increase in pituitary LH-RH reserve. Moreover, the amplitude of LH increase in response to LH-RH is generally proportional to circulating oestradiol and oestrone levels.

The pituitary overproduction of LH stimulates an increased secretion of androgens by the ovaries: testosterone and, mostly, androstenedione. These androgens can induce hirsutism, as discussed previously, and they also contribute to maintaining oestrogen production by peripheral conversion of androstenedione to oestrone and eventually to oestradiol (Grodin et al. 1973). A relatively high concentration of oestrogen in the pituitary results, provoking in turn an increase in the pituitary response to endogenous LH-RH, with a subsequent LH hypersecretion. A "vicious circle" is thus accomplished (Rebar et al. 1976; Yen et al. 1976) (Fig. 22). On the other hand, the rather low pituitary secretion of FSH could be responsible for an insufficient follicular maturation in this syndrome, the suppression of the preovulatory peak in estradiol, and therefore the absence of ovulation.

What is the primum mobile in this vicious circle? Is it a primary pituitary hypersensitivity to circulating oestrogens inducing a high pulse of LH, hyperstimulation of the ovarian stroma, and androgen overproduction? Could it be a hypersecretion of LH-RH by the hypothalamus? Due to technical problems this remains to be proved. Another hypothesis would be a primary defect in FSH secretion. There are good reasons in support of this latter mechanism.

When Short and London (1961) found exceedingly high concentrations of androstenedione but no oestrogens in the follicular fluid of polycystic ovaries, they concluded, as other authors (Axelrod and Goldzieher 1961), that polycystic ovaries have a defect in aromatase activity. Nevertheless, the mechanism of this abnormal ovarian steroidogenesis remained to be established.

Studies in rats (Dorrington et al. 1975; Erickson and Hsueh 1978) and humans (Moon et al. 1978) have shown that FSH plays a crucial role in stimulating ovarian oestrogen secretion by acting directly on the granulosa cells to increase aromatase enzyme activity. In view of defining a functional relationship between the reduced FSH to LH ratio in patients with polycystic ovaries and the decreased ability of such ovaries to secrete oestrogens, Erickson et al. (1979) examined the effects of FSH on polycystic ovaries. Granulosa cells obtained from medium-sized follicles of women with polycystic ovaries have little, if any, aromatase enzyme activity; however, they are capable of aromatization in vitro when appropriately stimulated with FSH. Similarly, administration of human FSH to patients with polycystic ovaries results in a rapid and dramatic increase in circulating oestradiol levels. These findings are

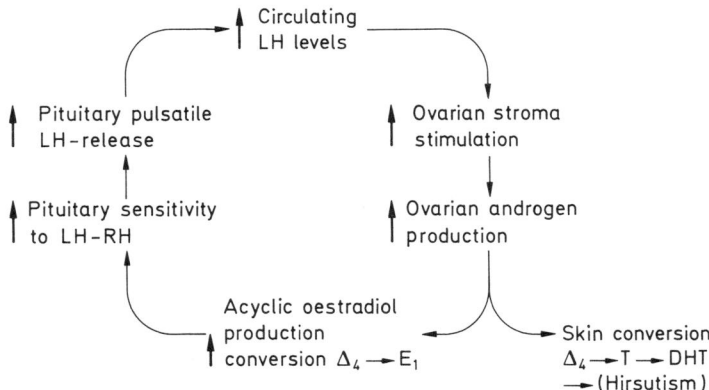

Fig. 22. Pathophysiology of polycystic ovary syndrome type I (from Yen et al. 1976)

consistent with the observation by other authors that polycystic ovaries are highly sensitive to exogenous FSH stimulation (Crooke et al. 1963; Jewelewicz et al. 1971).

Thus, granulosa cells from patients with polycystic ovaries have an inherent ability to respond to the FSH induction of aromatase activity. However, the Graafian follicles never develop to the size at which the aromatase enzyme normally becomes active. Such data suggest that in polycystic ovaries arrested follicle growth may be caused by a defect in quality and/or quantity of available FSH; thus folliculogenesis ceases at the mid-antral stage, and oestradiol is secreted in an insufficient amount to sensibilize granulosa cells to circulating FSH (Wilson et al. 1979) and to reach the preovulatory oestradiol peak which conditions the LH surge. As a result, the woman becomes anovulatory.

8. Treatment

The treatment of hirsutism due to the polycystic ovarian syndrome consists of blocking the ovarian overproduction of androgens with inhibitors of the gonadotropin secretion. This may be obtained by the use of oestrogen-progestagen preparations (see also Chap. L).

9. Conclusion

Although the pathophysiology of the polycystic ovarian syndrome has not been completely elucidated, the biochemical mechanism of this disease is now clearer. Indeed, no other case of amenorrhoea or spaniomenorrhoea, with or without hirsutism, is associated with high LH, normal or low FSH, and plasma androstenedione twice as high as normal. This association is seen neither in gonadotropic insufficiencies of hypothalamo-pituitary origin, nor in primary ovarian insufficiency; neither can it be found in other cases of hirsutism. An accidental preovulatory LH surge may be easily checked by several routine assays at various intervals. The dramatic response to LH-RH and the positive reaction to clomiphene citrate, which contributes not only the diagnosis but also to therapy, complete the current biochemical definition of the polycystic ovarian syndrome.

II. Virilizing Ovarian Tumours

The normal ovary synthesizes androgens, but most of these androgens are only precursors for oestrogen biosynthesis; only a small fraction is secreted as such.

Virilizing ovarian tumours produce large amounts of active androgens which induce intense clinical virilization. These tumours are original in several aspects. In addition to the quantitative increase in androgen secretion, a qualitative change in androgen biosynthesis and production occurs with a preferential secretion of testosterone. Ovarian tumours all develop from cells of the medulla of the primitive gonad, with three possibilities: they may derive from cells with androgen potential (rete ovarii, hilus cells), from cells with loss of aromatization potential, or from ectopic adrenal remnants, issued, like the ovarian medulla, from the central part of the mesonephric blastema.

These tumours remain difficult to classify and the best solution is still to do so according to pathological characteristics (Scully 1963; Mauvais-Jarvis et al. 1971; Novak and Woodruff 1974; Sternberg and Dhurandar 1977).

1. Pathological Classification

Ovarian virilizing tumours develop from a primitive gonad with multiple differentiation capacity (Morris and Scully 1958; Witschi 1963). There are three types of cells (cortex, medulla, and germ cells) and two possible sex orientations (male or female).

In the ovary, germ cells become ovogonia, the cortical cells become granulosa cells, and the medulla provides stroma and theca cells, whereas, in the testes, germ cells become spermatogonia, and cortical cells become Sertoli cells. The medulla provides the Leydig cells. From a pathological point of view, ovarian virilizing tumours may be divided into four main groups:

        Male-type tumours
        Female-type tumours
        Mixed tumours
        Functioning stroma tumours.

a) Arrhenoblastoma

This is the most frequent and typical of virilizing tumour because it is issued from the rete ovarii which reproduces the rete testis in the ovarian hilus. It consists of Sertoli and Leydig cells, and it has all the characteristics of testicular function: pathology, histo-enzymology, biosynthesis and secretion. Macroscopically, it is generally a large tumour, often solid but sometimes cystic with necrotic and haemorrhagic areas. Histologically, it consists of both Sertoli and Leydig cells in varying combinations and degrees of differentiation.

b) Hilus Cell Tumours

Rare and very small, this tumour develops in the hilus region from the cells described by Berger as "Leydig cells of the ovary". Very close to Leydig cells it actually contains Reinke crystalloids and lipochrome pigments and has a perineural disposition.

c) Lipid Cell Tumours

This unspecific term expresses the uncertainties concerning the origin of these tumours (Lipsett et al. 1970; Bonaventura et al. 1978; Adashi et al 1979) and designates tumours with large polyhedral cells which resemble adrenocortical or luteal cells.

Certain lipid cell tumours are thought to be Leydig cells because they have a perineural disposition and some Reinke crystalloids. Others appear to be related to adrenocortical cells since they are found in the hilus or the large ligament preferential location of adrenal remnants and because they are made up of pale cells in an adrenal glomerular or fascicular disposition. Lastly, they have been said to originate from luteinized stroma, because they are located in the cortex and are associated with clusters of luteinized stroma cells elsewhere in the cortex.

d) Granulosa and Theca Cell Tumours

Female-type cell tumours may be associated with clinical and biological hyperandrogenism, raising many questions: Are they so undifferentiated that Leydig or theca cells cannot be distinguished? Could female-type cells coexist with male-type cells that have remained unnoticed? Is a reactional luteinization of the stroma responsible or have these oestrogenic endocrine cells lost their aromatization capacity?

e) Gonadoblastomas

These tumours occur almost exclusively in intersexual states and are a good illustration of various possibilities of the primitive gonad since they associate germ cells, sex cords and primitive mesenchyma (Garvin et al. 1976; Govan et al. 1977).

f) Functional Stroma Tumours

Certain supposed non-functional tumours are sometimes associated with clinical signs of virilization. They may be benign (Brenner tumours, pseudomucinous cystadenomas) or malignant — adenocarcinomas and gastric metastases: so-called Krukenberg tumours (Ances and Ganis 1968)—. Usually a luteinized ovarian stroma is found and is completely different from the stroma of the tumour. This hyperplasia of the ovarian stroma could be induced by the tumour.

g) Luteoma

First described by Sternberg and Barclay in 1966, this "multinodular lipid cell formation", affecting both ovaries, occurs during pregnancy. Sometimes revealed by virilization of the mother during pregnancy or by pseudohermaphroditism of a female neonate, luteoma is often latent, as shown by the unexpected frequency in the case of laparotomy performed at the end of pregnancy (1 of 400 cases).

This tumour appears during pregnancy and disappears after delivery. It is not neoplastic in spite of its twisted aspect and, too often, in the course of a caesarean delivery, surgeons perform a hasty bilateral ovariectomy on seeing the two enormous masses resulting from overstimulation of the ovarian stroma by the large amounts of gonadotropin secreted during pregnancy. The histologic aspect is that of luteinized thecal hyperplasia and this "tumour" has therefore been called "pseudotumoral thecomatosis" (Laffargue et al. 1968; Shuster and Leake 1968; Polansky et al. 1975).

2. Steroidogenesis

Current data concerning steroidogenesis have been obtained from isolation of androgens in tumoral tissue and from incubations of tumour slices with radioactive tracers. In addition, gradient studies between ovarian and peripheral veins have completed the knowledge of ovarian biosynthesis.

These tumours, probably due to a dedifferentiation phenomenon, currently recover all the biosynthetic and secretory properties of the primitive gonad. The biosynthetic pathways observed and the steroids produced grossly depend on the histological type of tumour. However, no absolute relationship can be defined. The resulting secreted androgens are essentially active compounds, but qualitative and quantitative variations are possible.

a) Arrhenoblastoma

Wiest et al. (1959) showed that progesterone, when incubated with tumoral tissue, was converted into 17-hydroxyprogesterone and androstenedione, and Savard et al. (1961) isolated 17- and 20-hydroxylated metabolites of progesterone in addition to androstenedione and testosterone. Nevertheless, as for testes, it is no longer certain that this pathway is the only one in arrhenoblastoma. Kase and Conrad (1964) have, indeed, postulated that both Δ_5 and Δ_4 pathways may take place in these tumours, with a preponderance of Δ_5 pathway. Moreover, arrhenoblastoma seems capable of utilizing dehydroisoandrosterone sulphate as a substrate to be converted into androstenedione and testosterone. (Sandberg et al. 1966) This is of interest since such tumours may have an important sulphatase activity, and since the circulating level of dehydroisoandrosterone sulphate is generally elevated.

The main characteristic of arrhenoblastoma steroidogenesis consists in the capacity for producing testosterone (Kase and Conrad 1964), which has been demonstrated by incubation experiments with androstenedione or dehydroisoandrosterone as precursors, and by arterio-venous catheterizations. In the normal ovary, the ratio of plasma testosterone in ovarian over peripheral vein is around 5.0. In arrhenoblastoma this ratio reaches 40 (Mahesh et al. 1970). Likewise, the ratio of androstenedione over testosterone in the ovarian vein, which is normally around 20 in normal females, is lower than 1.0 in patients with arrhenoblastoma. Concerning the oestrogen production of arrhenoblastoma, it seems that, in spite of clinical symptoms of defeminization, a persistent oestrogenic effect is histologically observed in endometrial biopsies. This might be due either to a direct secretion by the tumour (Sato et al. 1969) or to peripheral conversion of secreted androgens.

b) Hilus Cell Tumours

In these tumours, androgen biosynthesis occurs through both Δ_5 and Δ_4 biosynthetic pathways. As in arrhenoblastoma, testosterone is the main androgen secreted (Jeffcoate and Prunty 1968). Dehydroisoandrosterone sulphate might also be a precursor for testosterone (Fahmy et al. 1968).

c) Luteoma

Steroid extraction of this tumour indicates a particularly high proportion of testosterone (O'Malley et al. 1967). Incubation studies have demonstrated that Δ_5 and Δ_4 pathways might be utilized for androgen biosynthesis. Androstenedione is the main product of the Δ_4 pathway and testosterone is essentially formed through the Δ_5 pathway which is predominant.

3. Clinical Features

Virilizing tumours are rare; they occur less frequently than feminizing tumours with a ratio of approximately 1:5. These tumors may be observed at all ages; however, arrhenoblastoma, the most frequent tumour, usually occurs in young women in their twenties.

From a clinical point of view, a virilizing ovarian tumour should always be suspected in the case of rapid dramatic virilization associated with signs of defeminization. The latter consist of oligomenorrhoea rapidly becoming amenorrhoea in women with previously normal cycles, and breast atrophy. In such tumours, major hirsutism with seborrhoea and acne is associated with changes in the voice, which deepens; changes in musculature, which becomes of the male-type; and, in the external genitalia characterized by a clitorial hypertrophy.

Clinical examination is considerably helpful when pelvic examination reveals an enlargement of one of the ovaries, but it cannot always detect an ovarian tumour which is often small.

4. Hormonal Investigations

a) Assays in Basal Conditions

The determination of urinary 17-ketosteroids is not helpful in the case of virilizing ovarian tumours. Even when these tumours secrete large amounts of active androgens, they may remain normal or be included in the higher values of the normal ranges. The determination of plasma testosterone is essential for the diagnosis. Currently, values higher than 2 ng/ml are observed. Plasma androstenedione is generally higher than 6 ng/ml; its level seems to be related to plasma testosterone concentration. Plasma oestradiol is generally in the normal range, sometimes elevated due to hepatic conversion of androgens into oestrogens.

b) Dynamic Tests

Suppressive tests using dexamethasone and stimulative tests with HCG or ACTH are not always reliable in determining the site and mechanism of the androgen oversecretion. Paradoxical responses are not uncommon. For example, dexamethasone may significantly reduce the level of plasma androgens in women with documented excess of ovarian production (Kirschner and Jacobs 1971). Ovarian tumours have been noted to be responsive to ACTH (Gallagher et al. 1962), whereas HCG may stimulate certain adrenal tumours (Werk et al. 1973; Givens et al. 1974). In addition, ovarian tumours, which are expected to be autonomous, sometimes respond to stimulation with HCG (Sato et al. 1969). An ovarian inhibition test using an oestrogen-progestagen combination may be proposed when the ovarian origin of hirsutism has been established. Its purpose is to distinguish between suppressible androgen secretion due to ovarian dystrophies, and non-suppressible tumoral secretion. However, this test demands an inhibition period of 1 month, which means wasting precious time. Moreover, it is not entirely specific since secretion of certain virilizing tumours can be partially suppressed (Gallagher et al. 1962), whereas in certain types of ovarian dystrophy, such as hyperthecosis, it cannot always be!

Theoretically, laparoscopy should help identify the virilizing tumour, but in reality, ovarian tumours cannot always be visualized with laparoscopy because they are often very small and sometimes only discovered on ovariotomy!

c) Other Methods for Diagnosis

Pelvic *echography* and/or *scanning* (Photopulos et al. 1979) can help diagnosis by defining the anatomic site of the tumour and also its size and extent. However, results are not always very clear-cut.

If there are good reasons to suspect a virilizing tumour (rapid clinical virilization, plasma testosterone concentration ≥ 2 ng/ml), the primary complementary examination to be carried out is catheterization of the gonadal and adrenal veins, with samplings for measurement of plasma testosterone and androstenedione. Androgen concentrations observed in gonadal veins are then compared to those noted in peripheral veins (Kirschner et al. 1976a; Weiland et al. 1978). This investigation is most interesting, although technical difficulties due to variations in ovarian vein anatomy, have made this procedure controversial (Wentz et al. 1976). An elevated androgen gradient *on one side* is a good indication of an abnormal ovarian secretion (Table 9). In addition, a low ratio of androstenedione to testosterone in the ovarian vein is a good argument for the tumoral origin of the androgen oversecretion. The sampling may be associated with venography. After the blood sample is obtained, a radiocontrast product may be injected for visualization of the expected ovarian tumour.

5. Differential Diagnosis

The sudden occurrence of virilization and amenorrhoea in a woman with previously normal menstrual cycles should immediately suggest a virilizing tumour. This may be confirmed by a high plasma testosterone concentration. Laparoscopy, pneumo-retroperitoneum, and catheterization of the efferent veins then distinguish between ovarian and adrenal origin of the tumour when clinical examination is insufficient.

If onset is less sudden, or if the woman's cycles were already abnormal, two other diagnosis could be suspected: a polycystic ovarian syndrome and a delayed onset congenital adrenal hyperplasia. In polycystic ovarian disease, both ovaries are theoretically increased, plasma testosterone does not exceed 1.0 ng/ml and plasma LH increases dramatically after LH-RH stimulation. By contrast, in patients with ovarian tumours, plasma LH is generally low and FSH is in the low normal range (Parker et al. 1974; Givens et al. 1974). In fact the diagnosis is not always so simple. Arrhenoblastoma may secondarily induce a polycystic ovarian syndrome (Zourias and Jones 1969) and, as a result, the clinical and hormonal features of the ovarian tumour, at least at the beginning of its evolution, may be misleading.

Diagnosis is easier in the case of delayed onset congenital adrenal hyperplasia, since the increase in precursors above the enzymatic defect may be easily determined in basal conditions and particularly after ACTH stimulation of the adrenals.

6. Prognosis

The prognosis of endocrine ovarian tumours is generally more favourable than that of non-secreting tumours. Malignancy is estimated at 20%. The histological type,

Table 9. Differences in plasma testosterone of ovarian vein (V) and artery (A) (from Simmer, in discussion of Mahesh and Greenblatt 1964)

Ovary	Δ(V-A) Testosterone (μg/100 ml)
Normal	0.09
Polycystic	0.37
Arrhenoblastoma	9.95

the degree of differentiation and, above all, whether the tumour is localized in one ovary or has extended to neighbouring organs, determine individual prognosis. Nevertheless, virilizing tumours have a particularly good prognosis with localized and slow evolution and very few rare and late metastases.

7. Treatment

Malignancy potential being slight, operative therapy could be limited to salpingo-ovariectomy in young women with unilateral ovarian tumours without extension to neighbouring organs, in order to preserve fertility (Novak and Long 1965). Conservative surgery should only be performed following a rigorous examination of the contralateral ovary and regular check-up in women over 40. However, it is safer to perform bilateral ovariectomy and total hysterectomy if laparotomy reveals extension to the contralateral ovary and to neighbouring organs. Surgery must be as widespread as possible and completed by postoperative cobalt therapy or chemotherapy.

Following removal of the tumour, a rapid clinical improvement ensues: the menstrual cycle becomes rapidly ovulatory. Young women become capable of having normal pregnancies and if the diagnosis is early enough, hirsutism significantly regresses. However, when surgery is performed late and virilization has set in for a long time, it persists irreversibly in spite of improvement of the other symptoms.

8. Conclusion

Virilizing ovarian tumours are rare causes of hirsutism. They reproduce all types of primitive gonad cells and show great variety in steroid biosynthesis; however, secretion of an active androgen, testosterone, predominates. The resulting intense virilization often permits early diagnosis; this, added to the fact that such tumours have a weak malignancy potential, makes their prognosis favourable.

The difficulty in visualizing these tumours before surgery emphasizes the importance of catheterization techniques. Differential diagnosis with polycystic ovarian syndrome, particularly at the beginning of tumoral evolution, must be based on well-documented clinical and biological data.

III. Ovarian Hyperthecosis

The so-called hyperthecosis, thecomatosis and stromal thecosis (Fraenkel 1943; Culiner and Shippel 1949) have often been assimilated to virilizing ovarian tumours because of the intensity of the stromal and thecal hyperplasia (Scully 1963),with islands of luteinized thecal cells in the stroma at a distance from follicles, and because of the severity of the virilization syndrome. However, hyperthecosis is a benign disease and it seems to be much closer to polycystic ovarian syndrome type I.

Both diseases are characterized by hirsutism associated with important menstrual disorders: oligomenorrhoea or amenorrhoea. However in hyperthecosis, hirsutism is more pronounced and associated with other signs of virilization. The androgen overproduction is greater than in polycystic ovarian syndrome (Bardin et al. 1967; Judd et al. 1973; Abraham and Burster 1976; Braithwaite 1979) and is qualitatively different from that of the polycystic ovarian syndrome. Plasma testosterone and androstenedione levels are often similar to those observed in ovarian tumours with a male-type pattern. The androstenedione/testosterone ratio in the ovarian veins, which is normally around 20 both in normal women and in patients with polycystic ovarian syndrome, was found to be lower than 1.0 in a case of ovarian hyperthecosis (Bardin et al. 1967). The production rate of plasma oestrone is greater than in polycystic ovarian syndrome, as might be expected because of the higher production rates of androgens (Aiman et al. 1978). Plasma FSH level is normal, whereas LH may be elevated (Karam and Hajj 1979), but this observation has been inconsistently noted. Hyperthecosis ovaries fail to respond to the usual treatment of anovulation proposed in the polycystic ovarian syndrome, in particular to clomiphene citrate administration.

Genetic factors have been suggested in the transmission of this affection (Givens et al. 1971; Judd et al. 1973); the hypothesis of an enzymatic block has also been raised, and the possible pathogenetic role of the LH abnormality remains to be explored.

The treatment of ovarian hyperthecosis is based on suppression of ovarian overproduction by oestrogen-progestagen combinations (Bardin et al. 1967). However, this treatment often proves inconclusive. In such patients, one must sometimes resort to bilateral ovariectomy, because of the inconsistent success of the cuneiform resection (Givens et al. 1971; Karam and Hajj 1979).

K. Idiopathic Hirsutism

Based on the androgen action mechanism (Fig. 23), hirsutism may result from two factors: (1) an oversecretion of virilizing androgens either from the ovaries or the adrenal glands, or (2) a hypersensitivity of the target cells in the skin to circulating androgens, that is, *idiopathic hirsutism*.

Idiopathic hirsutism is a good illustration of a new approach to endocrinology, namely, *receptivity*. The pathophysiology of secretion itself has become relatively easy to control, whether excessive or absent, by suppressive or substitutive therapy. Research is now currently oriented towards target organs — their receptivity and their regulation (Verhoeven and Wilson 1979). Regarding androgens, the hypersensitivity of the skin to these hormones might be responsible for idiopathic hirsutism, whereas insensitivity is responsible for the testicular feminization syndrome (Griffin and Wilson 1980; Kuttenn et al. 1979 a, 1980 a).

I. Basis of Androgen Hypersensitivity

The theory has been advanced that hirsutism may be a manifestation of increased end-organ sensitivity to normal androgen levels and is based on the obvious differences in the rate of development of hirsutism in women receiving testosterone (Kennedy et al. 1953). This theory was further supported by the occurence of normal plasma testosterone levels in several studies of hirsute women (Dignam et al. 1964; Korenman et al. 1965; Lloyd et al. 1966), and by a better understanding of the action mechanism of androgens on target cells.

The pilosebaceous gland is a key androgen target organ since all the biochemical events involved in androgen activity in male accessory organs have been described at this site (Fig. 23). Testosterone enters cells as free testosterone and is reduced to its active metabolite, dihydrotestosterone, by a specific enzyme 5α-reductase (Voigt et

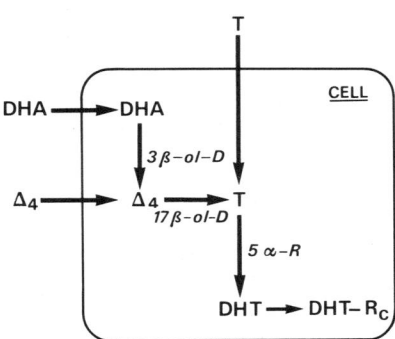

Fig. 23. A general scheme of "utilization" by human skin of plasmactive and -inactive androgens. *DHA*, dehydroisoandrosterone; Δ_4, androstenedione; *T*, testosterone; *3β-ol-D*, 3β-hydroxysteroid dehydrogenase; *17β-ol-D*, 17β-hydroxysteroid dehydrogenase; *5α-R*, 5α-reductase; R_C, receptor; *DHT*, dehydrotestosterone

al. 1970). Dihydrotestosterone binds its specific cytosolic receptor (Keenan et al. 1974; Griffin et al. 1976), and the dihydrotestosterone receptor complex is then transferred into the nucleus (Amrhein et al. 1976; Collier et al. 1978). Moreover, it is known that human skin is capable of converting dehydroisoandrosterone and especially androstenedione into testosterone and dihydrotestosterone (Gomez and Hsia 1968; Flamigni et al. 1971). The skin thus appears to participate not only in the catabolism of androgens but also in the formation of active androgens from inactive precursors supplied through the blood.

II. Hypersensitivity Versus Androgen Overproduction

By definition, idiopathic hirsutism should not be accompanied by an increased androgen secretion. The hyperstimulation of the cutaneous androgen target cells (essentially the pilosebaceous complex) should be the result of an abnormality in the reception of the androgenic message. For these reasons, idiopathic hirsutism long remained a diagnosis of exclusion, and the denomination of "idiopathic" was reserved for cases of hirsutism not accompanied by the abnormalities suggestive of adrenal or ovarian overproduction.

However, numerous studies have been carried out to examine the respective roles of overproduction of active androgens and skin hypersensitivity to circulating androgens in idiopathic hirsutism. Bardin and Lipsett (1967) were the first to show that testosterone and androstenedione blood production rates were higher in patients with idiopathic hirsutism than in normal women, even though they were lower than in polycystic ovarian syndrome. Plasma androstenedione was also found to be significantly higher than normal in patients with idiopathic hirsutism. It increases in proportion to its production rate, since its metabolic clearance rate remains the same in all cases. Plasma testosterone was higher than in normal women, but the ranges overlapped in contrast to production rate, which did not; moreover, the testosterone metabolic clearance rate of hirsute women is significantly higher than that of normal women. Bardin and Lipsett (1967) therefore suggested that the testosterone metabolic rate may vary directly with "some function of testosterone production" and they evoked the role of TeBG. The same results have been further detailed in a large group of patients by Kirschner and Bardin (1972).

In more recent studies, Kirschner et al. (1976 b) demonstrated frequent secretory abnormalities occurring in idiopathic hirsutism. These observations were obtained from the simultaneous measurement of androgens in the peripheral venous blood and in venous blood obtained by retrograde catheterization of the ovarian and adrenal veins (Kirschner and Jacobs 1971). These studies pointed out that most cases of such androgen hypersecretion were of ovarian origin and that hypersecretion of adrenal origin was extremely rare. This was contrary to opinions previously stated (Mahesh et al. 1964; Casey et al. 1966; Casey and Nabarro 1967).

In practice, there are essentially two androgens involved in the stimulation of the pilosebaceous receptor:
1) *Testosterone* not bound to TeBG, either directly secreted or produced (60%) by peripheral transformation of androstenedione (Rosenfeld 1971; Clark et al. 1975; Vermeulen and Ando 1979; Moll and Rosenfield 1979).

2) *Circulating androstenedione*, which is the main androgen secreted in women and which is more often found elevated in idiopathic hirsutism than testosterone itself. It can be reduced to testosterone in the pilosebaceous receptor, but this testosterone will never appear in the plasma.

The raised metabolic clearance rate of testosterone in hirsutism reported by Bardin and Lipsett (1967) supports the theory of the increased "utilization" of androgens. It results mainly from an increased metabolism of testosterone by extrahepatic tissues. This is shown by the higher rate of conversion of testosterone to dihydrotestosterone and 3α-androstanediol in the blood of hirsute women than in that of normal women (Mahoudeau et al. 1971). This increased metabolic clearance rate of testosterone is facilitated by the low concentration of TeBG in the plasma of hirsute patients (Dray et al. 1968 a; Vermeulen et al. 1969) and by a higher than normal concentration of unbound testosterone (Clark et al. 1971; Rosenfield, 1971). Vermeulen and Ando (1979) recently emphasized that the testosterone metabolic clearance rate was linearly related to both the free and non-specifically bound testosterone fractions of the plasma.

TeBG binding affinity and capacity are themselves functions of testosterone production and action at the hepatic level, since its level is higher in normal women than in normal men. It is known to increase under the effect of oestrogen and to decrease under androgen stimulation (Vermeulen et al. 1969; Kirschner and Bardin 1972; Vermeulen and Ando 1979; Moll and Rosenfield 1979).

However, low plasma TeBG, increased plasma free testosterone and increased androgen metabolic clearance are only indirect data which suggest that a hypersensitivity of androgen target cells to circulating hormone exists! In vivo data do not provide evidence that an increase in the utilization of androgens by the cutaneous receptor exists in idiopathic hirsutism. The proof can only be provided by carrying out in vivo and in vitro studies in parallel. Such studies should assess, on the one hand, the metabolism of testosterone in the cutaneous receptor of hirsute women and, on the other hand, circulating and excreted androgens which reflect either the production or the peripheral metabolism of the male hormones.

III. Clinical and Biological Characteristics

Idiopathic hirsutism shows no clinical differences from other types of hirsutism. It should be noted, however, that it is not associated with any other sign of hyperandrogenism (Kirschner et al. 1976b) concerning virilization of the external genital area, male-type muscle development, deep voice, etc. Menstrual cycles remain regular and ovulatory (Kuttenn et al. 1977). The patients are often of Mediterranean origin.

Whatever the type of hirsutism, the same procedure should be followed: is it due to overproduction or hypersensitivity?

1. Criteria for Estimation of Androgen Production (Table 10)

The estimation of plasma levels of testosterone and androstenedione reliably reflects active androgen production. This is particularly true for androstenedione, the metabolic clearance rate of which remains constant in all the subjects.

Table 10. Biological criteria for assessment of idiopathic hirsutism

Plasma	Testosterone Androstenedione Dehydroisoandrosterone sulphate?	Androgen Production
Plasma dihydrotestosterone Urinary 3α-androstanediol Skin 5α-reductase activity (in vitro determination)		Androgen "utilization" by skin

2. Criteria for Estimation of Peripheral Androgen Consumption (Table 10)

Dihydrotestosterone and 3α-androstanediol are potent androgens not directly secreted by the gonads or the adrenals. Dihydrotestosterone originates essentially from the 5α-reduction of testosterone and androstenedione in the hepatic and extrahepatic tissues (Mahoudeau et al. 1971; Ito and Horton). 3α-Androstanediol appears to have the same origin. However, the different studies carried out on the origin of dihydrotestosterone and plasma 3α-androstanediol, as well as of urinary 3α-androstanediol, do not permit definition of a distinction between the synthesis of these steroids occurring, on the one hand, in the liver and, on the other hand in the target organs. Therefore the in vitro assessment of the capacity of "sexual" skin to metabolize testosterone to dihydrotestosterone and 3α-androstanediol seems the most accurate method of determining the actual degree of androgen "utilization" of dihydrotestosterone by target cells.

3. Personal Data

According to these criteria, a study was carried out on 40 hirsute women aged 14 to 40 years compared with 20 normal women and 20 normal men of equivalent age (Kuttenn et al. 1977; Mauvais-Jarvis et al. 1979). Only 20 patients presented an idiopathic hirsutism on the basis of purely clinical criteria (absence of menstrual disorders or signs of hypercorticism, etc.). In 14 cases, hirsutism was due to polycystic ovarian syndrome with anovulatory cycles, enlarged ovaries being found upon clinical examination and/or laparoscopy. In six cases, hirsutism was of adrenal origin (three Cushing and three congenital adrenal hyperplasia). These patients were investigated in vivo by measuring testosterone and dihydrotestosterone in the plasma, and urinary 3α-androstanediol (Wright et al, 1978). In addition, 5α-reductase activity was measured in vitro in 150 mg samples of pubic skin obtained under local anesthesia as described previously (Mauvais-Jarvis et al. 1974).

a) In Vivo Studies

Plasma testosterone was sligthly higher in women with idiopathic hirsutism than in normal women (51.0 ± 22 ng/dl compared to 33.2 ± 12.3 ng/dl), but this increase was not significant and the mean value was markedly below that observed in the cases of adrenal and ovarian hirsutism. However, plasma androstenedione concentration was elevated in most cases of idiopathic hirsutism (203 ± 100 ng/dl compared to

133 ± 30 ng/dl). Here also the observed values were lower than those in women with ovarian or adrenal virilism (Fig. 24).

On the other hand, although the concentration of dihydrotestosterone in women with idiopathic hirsutism was higher than in normal women, it did not differ from the values of the women with ovarian or adrenal virilism (Fig. 24).

The urinary excretion of androstanediol (Fig. 26) was much higher in women with idiopathic hirsutism than in normal women (88 ± 36 µg/24 h, compared to 36 ± 12 µg/24h), but not as much as that observed in the women with polycystic ovaries.

b) In Vitro Studies

The cutaneous 5α-reductase activity measured in vitro (Fig. 25) was markedly elevated in women with idiopathic hirsutism. The conversion of radioactive testosterone to dihydrotestosterone and androstanediol in these patients attained 205 ± 54 fmol/mg skin. This activity was comparable to that of normal men and differed significantly from that of the normal women. In addition, it was clearly superior to that seen in the other cases of hirsutism due to androgen overproduction: ovarian and even more, adrenal.

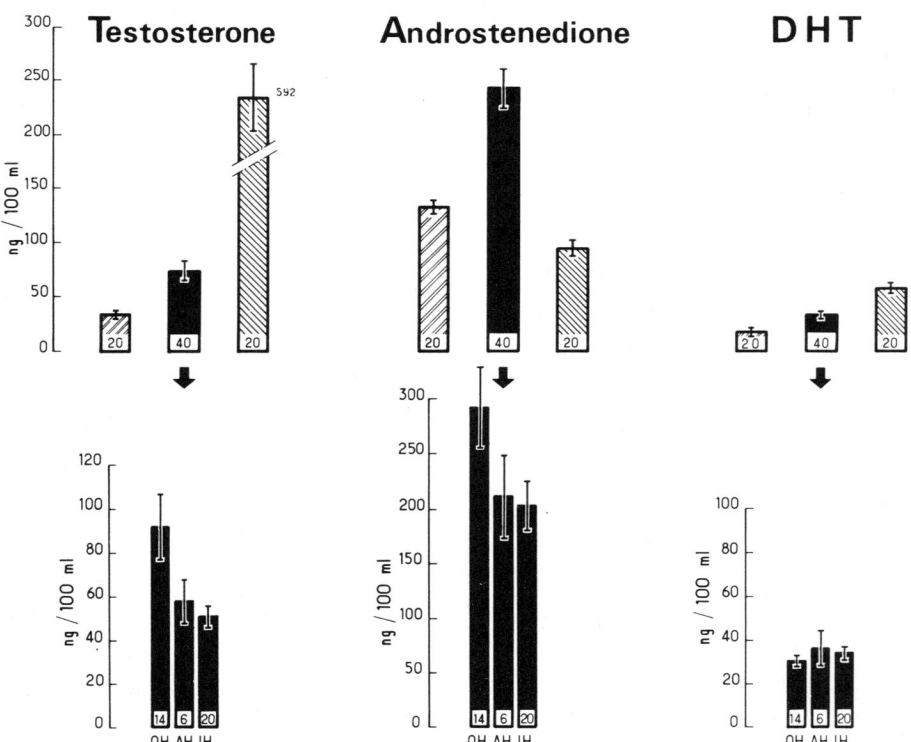

Fig. 24. Mean concentrations ($\pm$ SEM) of testosterone, androstenedione and dihydrotestosterone (*DHT*) in the plasma of 40 hirsute women (■), 20 normal women (▨) and 20 normal men (▩) and women in the three subgroups of hirsutism: ovarian (*OH*), adrenal (*AH*) and idiopathic (*IH*). The number of subjects studied is given at the base of each bar. Kuttenn et al. 1977

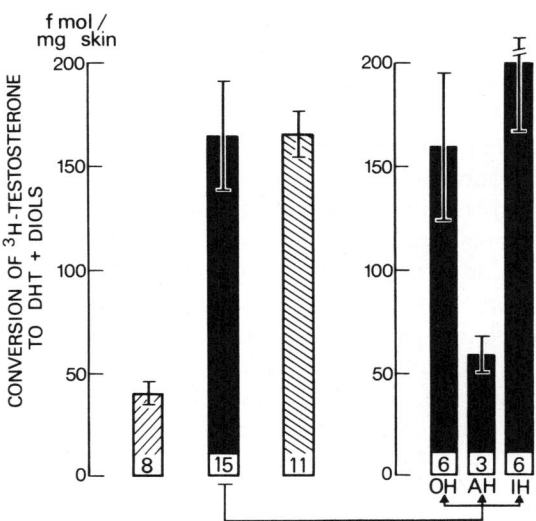

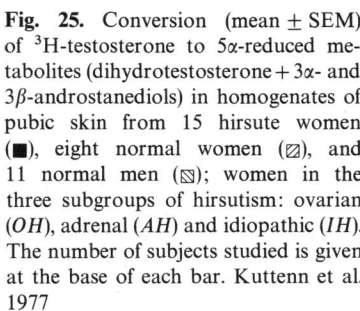

Fig. 25. Conversion (mean ± SEM) of ³H-testosterone to 5α-reduced metabolites (dihydrotestosterone + 3α- and 3β-androstanediols) in homogenates of pubic skin from 15 hirsute women (■), eight normal women (▨), and 11 normal men (▨); women in the three subgroups of hirsutism: ovarian (*OH*), adrenal (*AH*) and idiopathic (*IH*). The number of subjects studied is given at the base of each bar. Kuttenn et al. 1977

c) Interpretation of Results

These results suggest that the production of androgens, and particularly of androstenedione, is increased in idiopathic hirsutism (Fig. 26). This agrees with recently published data (Andre and James 1974; Kirschner et al. 1976b). The source of this overproduction of androstenedione could not have been brought to light by the classic dynamic tests. However, the only constant fact observed in our studies was the elevation in idiopathic hirsutism of testosterone and androstenedione after HCG (Mauvais-Jarvis and Kuttenn 1976b). This result agrees with the data obtained by Kirschner and Jacobs (1971), Kirschner and Bardin (1972) and Kirschner et al. (1976b). According to these authors, in idiopathic hirsutism there is an almost constant ovarian hypersecretion of testosterone and, especially, of

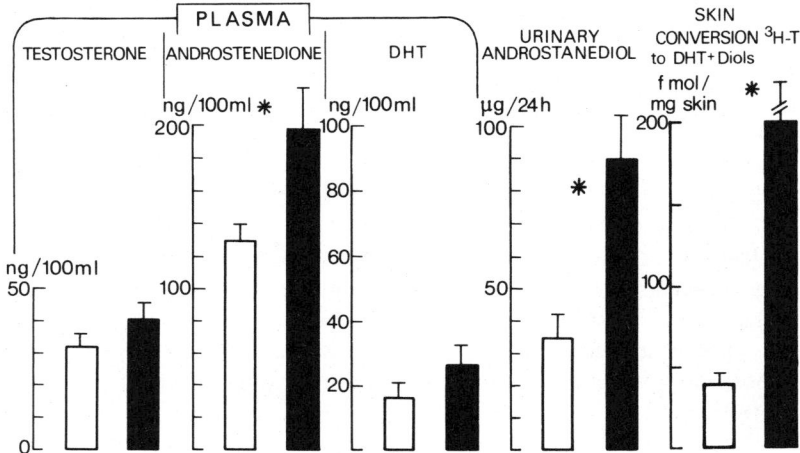

Fig. 26. Parameters of androgen production and skin utilization in women with idiopathic hirsutism. $P < 0.001$; □, normal women; ■, patients with idiopathic hirsutism (20 cases)

androstenedione even if the dexamethasone suppression of these plasma steroids suggests an adrenal origin.

As far as the parameters of peripheral "utilization" of androgens are concerned, it clearly appears that in idiopathic hirsutism urinary 3α-androstanediol is more significantly elevated than plasma dihydrotestosterone. The following explanation is proposed: the major part of the dihydrotestosterone synthesized in the target cells and the liver is reduced in situ to 3α-androstanediol and never appears in the circulation. The 3α-androstanediol is itself, for the most part, excreted in the urine. The level of production of 3α-androstanediol in the plasma may be calculated by multiplying the metabolic clearance of this steroid by its plasma concentration (Bird et al. 1974; Kinouchi and Horton 1974). The obtained value is very close to the daily excretion of 3α-androstanediol, at least in normal man. This statement substantiates the hypothesis that 3α-androstanediol is a final metabolic product of testosterone (Kuttenn et al. 1977).

Because androstenedione appears to be the principal source of dihydrotestosterone in women (Ito and Horton 1971), the elevated level of dihydrotestosterone observed in women with idiopathic hirsutism may be due to peripheral conversion of this prehormone. The highly increased excretion of 3α-androstanediol in these same women reflects at the same time a raised production of androstenedione and an increase in the peripheral conversion of this hormone. In fact, the level of production of androstenedione which is approximately 3.0 mg/24 h in the normal women, may increase to 8.0 mg/24 h in hirsute women (Bardin and Lipsett 1967). The contribution of androstenedione to urinary androstanediol was calculated after intravenous injection of radioactive androstenedione (Baulieu and Mauvais-Jarvis 1964) and increases from 0.5% in normal women to 1.0% in hirsute women (unpublished work). The variations of these two parameters may explain the considerable differences seen between normal and hirsute women (from 12 to 100 μg/24 h), as well as the variations of excretion within the group of hirsute women itself. The same calculations have been performed for the contribution of testosterone to urinary androstanediol. In hirsute women this does not exceed 20 μg/24 h.

The measurement of urinary 3α-androstanediol in women provides precise information on the peripheral metabolism of androstenedione. This seems important because, contrary to what may be observed for testosterone, an increase in the metabolism of androstenedione by the extrahepatic tissues is not reflected by an increase of the metabolic clearance rate of androstenedione. In idiopathic hirsutism the observed increase in plasma androstenedione reflects the secretion of this prehormone as reported by Kirschner et al. (1976 b). However, it seems reasonable to propose that the increase, in the skin itself, of the conversion of androstenedione to testosterone and then to dihydrotestosterone plays a major role in the appearance and maintenance of this hirsutism. In other words, the observation in these patients of an increased cutaneous 5α-reductase activity contrasting with the only moderately elevated levels of testosterone and androstenedione supports the hypothesis that there exists in idiopathic hirsutism an abnormality of the receptivity to androgens.

This hypersensitivity to androgens with an increase in their peripheral utilization has provided an explanation for the following biological data previously reported in idiopathic hirsutism:

1) Increased testosterone metabolic clearance rate (Bardin and Lipsett 1967);
2) High rate of blood conversion of testosterone to dihydrotestosterone and 3α-androstanediol (Mahoudeau et al. 1971);
3) Low TeBG level (Dray et al. 1968 a); and
4) increased concentration of unbound testosterone (Vermeulen 1969; Clark et al. 1975; Rosenfield 1971).

All these characteristics result from an increased androgen action especially in the liver, which acts as a target organ. In any case, the simultaneous determination of plasma androgens and of the capacity of the sexual skin to transform testosterone to its 5α-reduced metabolites appears necessary to us for the assessment of the respective roles of hormonal androgen secretion and exaggerated androgen "utilization" by the skin in the appearance of hirsutism.

The mechanism of androgen action and skin sensitivity also depends on the binding capacity and affinity of the dihydrotestosterone cytosol receptor (Kuttenn et al. 1979 a). Its absence and/or decrease is known to be responsible for androgen resistance syndrome, that is, male pseudohermaphroditism. The increase of cytosol androgen receptor capacity has been implicated in lesions such as seborrhoea and acne (Bonne et al. 1977). In hirsutism due to overproduction, no difference has been found between the levels of skin cytosol androgen receptor in patients and those in normal women (personal data). Idiopathic hirsutism due to primary increased androgen receptor capacity in the skin can be imagined, but remains to be demonstrated!

IV. Treatment

To be effective, treatment must be based on pathophysiological analysis. The battle can be led on two fronts: (1) suppression of androgen access to the cell and (2) inhibition of androgen action at the level of target cells. Actually, the only efficient treatments are those that act on both levels simultaneously (see Sect. L).

V. Conclusion

Androgen overproduction and skin hypersensitivity seem to be two distinct but eventually additive mechanisms:
1) An androgen overproduction has been demonstrated in certain cases of hirsutism, still considered as idiopathic, in the absence of obvious ovarian and adrenal dysfunction. In these cases, the mild androgen overproduction provides a substrate to the skin sensitivity system.
2) An increased testosterone production rate is not necessarily associated with hirsutism (Bardin and Lipsett 1967; Leichter and Jacobs 1976; Bouchard et al. 1981). The end-organ sensitivity and especially the potential induction of skin 5α-reductase under the oversecreted androgen stimulation is determinant in this instance.

When reviewing the literature, it is surprising to note the absence of rigorous criteria for the distribution of the label "idiopathic hirsutism", which is often used as a simple exclusion diagnosis in the absence of ovarian or adrenal abnormalities.

Cases of hirsutism are thus often filed under "idiopathic" even when two basic conditions are not met:
1) regular and ovulatory menstrual cycles (which should eliminate ovarian hirsutism), and
2) normal plasma 17-hydroxyprogesterone levels before and after stimulation by ACTH to eliminate delayed onset congenital adrenal hyperplasia which often clinically resembles idiopathic hirsutism. As for the supposed normal plasma testosterone level, it has been demonstrated that such a normal level does not necessarily imply a normal production rate.

Under the circumstances, it seems clear that "idiopathic" hirsutism, by definition, may no longer be considered as such, since it is often accompanied by a hypersecretion of androgens, in particular androstenedione, which may be concentrated in different sites (especially in the skin), the source of this oversecretion being essentially the ovary. However, one can imagine that a more rigorous selection of the patients would give rise to a hirsute patients group with only one abnormality, i.e. a disorder of receptivity. Indeed, the in vitro data obtained from the study of androgen metabolism in the skin of hirsute patients have provided a pathophysiological label for this frequent sort of hirsutism that no secretory abnormality alone could justify.

This abnormality is characterized essentially by the presence (congenital or acquired) of a markedly increased 5α-reductase activity, which permits the formation of dihydrotestosterone from free testosterone once it has crossed the cell membrane and, particularly, from circulating androstenedione having passively crossed the cellular barrier.

The excess of skin 5α-reductase activity is currently considered as a cause of hirsutism, but both the exact level of the abnormality in the regulation of the enzyme and its genetic control remain to be demonstrated.

L. Treatment of Hirsutism

I. Introduction

Because hirsutism results from either an androgen overproduction or from hypersensitivity of the skin to androgens, its treatment must therefore suppress the pathological processes involved in order to be effective.

Androgen overproduction, if any, must be suppressed by, e. g. surgery of ovarian or adrenal tumours, substitutive cortisol therapy in the case of congenital adrenal hyperplasia due to an enzymatic defect, or institution of ovarian gonadotropin stimulation in the case of polycystic ovaries or hyperthecosis.

Antiandrogens must be used as much as possible. They act on the target cell and inhibit the action of remaining circulating androgens. The anti-androgens currently used are progesterone and anti-androgenic progestogens.

II. Methods

1. Oestrogens

a) Mechanism of Action

Oestrogens are known to act at three different levels:
1) *In sufficient dosages*, they have a *negative feedback effect on gonadotropin secretion* and are thus able to suppress the stimulation by LH of the ovarian cortical stroma, which seems to be the principal source of ovarian androgens (Marsh et al. 1976).
2) *Oestrogens also increase the synthesis of TeBG*, thus reducing the amount of free circulating testosterone (Anderson 1976).
3) *Moreover, oestrogens are competitive inhibitors* of dihydrotestosterone at the level of the cytosolic receptor (Fang and Liao 1969; Baulieu and Jung 1970; Mangan and Mainwaring 1972).
4) Used on a long-term basis oestrogens also inhibit the cutaneous 5α-reductase activity (Kuttenn and Mauvais-Jarvis 1975). However, oestrogens may not be considered as competitive inhibitors of skin 5α-reductase (Voigt et al. 1970). One must therefore imagine an intracellular action of oestrogens at other sites of action, i.e. competition with the cytosolic protein or action on the nuclear material (Mangan et al. 1967) with degeneration of androgen-dependent or androgen-activating systems of synthesis, such as 5α-reductase, by a logic of competition not yet explained.

b) Clinical Use

Oestrogens are used in association with progestogens in combined, or more often sequential, oestrogen-progestogen "pills". Such associations are used for the treatment of hirsutism resulting from ovarian androgen overproduction and that resulting from skin hypersensitivity, known as "idiopathic hirsutism".

Figures 27 and 28 show the biological results of such a treatment in 20 cases of hirsutism of ovarian and idiopathic origin. A sequential preparation (Ovanon), was used (Mauvais-Jarvis et al. 1977). The treatment for one cycle consisted of 50 µg ethinyl-oestradiol alone for 8 days and the same dose associated with 2.5 mg lynestrenol daily for 14 days. This treatment resulted in a double effect. First, there was an antisecretory action which resulted in a marked decrease of plasma testosterone and androstenedione, and which was obtained after 1 month of treatment. Secondly, the action of oestrogen on the utilization of androgens in the target organs was supported partly by the decrease of plasma dihydrotestosterone and urinary 3α-androstanediol. However, part of the effect of these steroids might be attributed to the decreased overproduction of androstenedione. The spectacular drop in cutaneous 5α-reductase activity in vitro, observed after 12 months of treatment, constitutes a direct argument in favour of oestrogen action on the target cell. The treatment of hirsutism by synthetic oestrogens therefore seems justified, at least on biochemical grounds. Practically speaking, their efficacy is shown by (1) the normalization of plasma testosterone and androstenedione levels (Fig. 27) and urinary 3α-androstanediol secretion, following 2 months' treatment, (2) the decrease to normal of testosterone 5α-reductase activity in the skin after 12 months' treatment (Fig. 28), and (3) the decrease in hair thickness, density and removal frequency after several months' treatment.

Similar results have been reported by Givens et al. (1976 a). However, such a treatment is only effective in ovarian hirsutism where it can inhibit ovarian androgen overproduction. It is often disappointing in the treatment of idiopathic hirsutism! Moreover, oestrogen-progestogen associations have the same contraindications as synthetic oestrogens: hypertension, diabetes, hyperlipidaemia, obesity (see Sect. L.II.3 b).

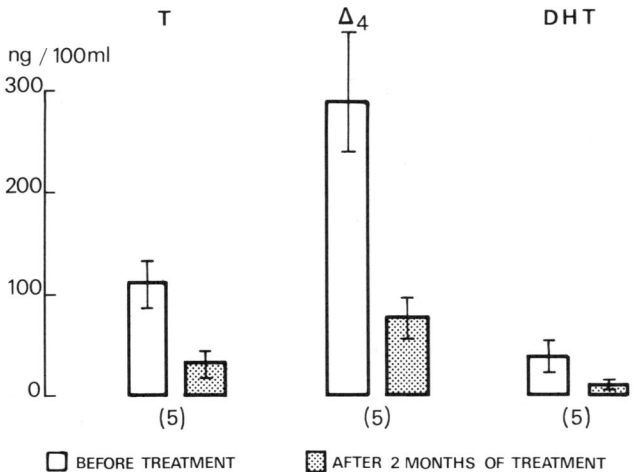

Fig. 27. Effect of an oestrogen-progestogen combination: Ovanon (see text for details) on plasma androgens in hirsute women. T, testosterone; Δ_4, androstenedione; DHT, dihydrotestosterone

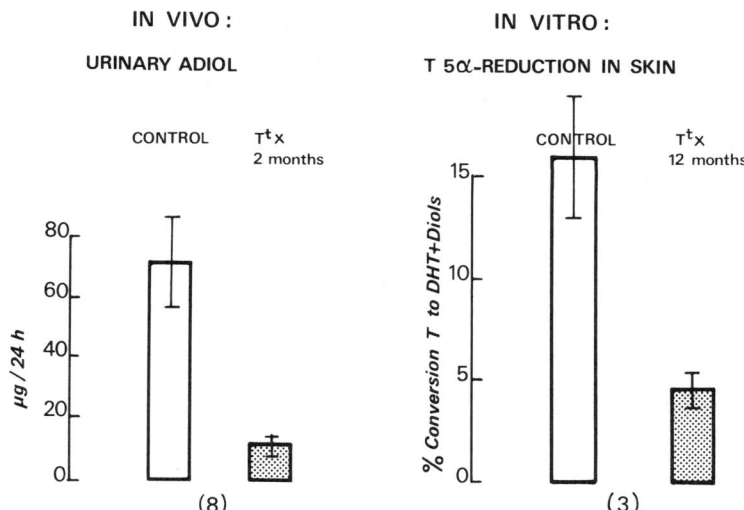

Fig. 28. Effect of an oestrogen-progestogen combination Ovanon (see text for details) on urinary 3α-androstanediol excretion (*Adiol*) and testosterone 5α-reduction into dihydrotestosterone and 3α- and 3β-androstanediols in pubic skin homogenates. $T^t \times 2\ months$, treatment for 2 months; $T^t \times 12\ months$, treatment for 12 months

2. Progesterone

Progesterone is a classic anti-androgen (Dorfman and Dorfman 1960; Lerner 1964; Dorfman 1967). It is generally considered as the best competitive inhibitor of testosterone 5α-reductase (Voigt et al. 1970; Massa and Martini 1971; Mauvais-Jarvis et al. 1974, 1976). Indeed, the 5α-reductase enzyme present in human skin has a greater affinity for progesterone than for testosterone (Fig. 29).

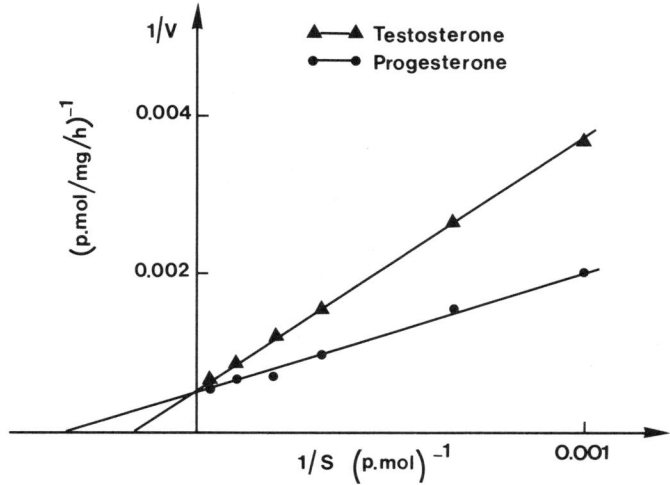

Fig. 29. Lineweaver-Burk plot of the apparition of 5α-reduced metabolites (dihydrotestosterone + androstanediols) from testosterone and progesterone as a function of substrate concentration in human pubic skin microsomes

In fact, progesterone acts as a competitive inhibitor at several levels of androgen action. It is not only an inhibitor of testosterone 5α-reductase, but also an inhibitor of dihydrotestosterone binding to the specific cytosolic receptor (Fang and Liao 1969; Baulieu and Jung 1970; Mangan and Mainwaring 1972; Wright et al. 1976, 1979, 1980). In addition, progesterone and its 5α-reduced metabolite, dihydroprogesterone, inhibits the 3α- and 3β-androstanediols (Wright et al. 1980; Giacomini and Wright 1980). However, progesterone has no antigonadotropic activity. Moreover, when administered orally, progesterone is extensively metabolized in the liver. It is therefore essentially used by percutaneous administration (Mauvais-Jarvis et al. 1974). Due to its merely local competitive action, it may be utilized in pathology which can be improved on a short-term basis, such as seborrhoea, acne etc. (Mauvais-Jarvis and Kuttenn 1973; Cherif-Cheikh and de Lignières 1974). It is not useful in disorders such as hirsutism, which demand long-term treatment; the hair growth cycle being 20 months long, whenever the slightest application is missed hair growth takes over. Progesterone is therefore only a complementary treatment for disorders of sebaceous gland activity, associated with hirsutism.

3. Cyproterone Acetate

a) Mechanism of Action

Cyproterone acetate (1,2α-methylene-6-chloro-pregna-4, 6-diene-17α–ol–3, 20-dione-1α-acetate) was first known as a progestin (Wiechert 1967). In 1963, its anti-androgenic properties were demonstrated in animals (Hamada et al. 1963). Cyproterone acetate acts as a competitive inhibitor of dihydrotestosterone, binding to its cytosol receptor (Neuman et al. 1970). In contrast to cyproterone, cyproterone acetate is not only a progestin and an anti-androgen compound, but also has an antigonadotropic effect (Neuman 1977).

The anti-androgen activity of cyproterone acetate was first successfully applied at a dose of 100–200 mg/day in hypersexual men (Lashet et al. 1967) and in cases of precocious puberty (Rager et al. 1973). Cyproterone acetate in association with ethinyl-oestradiol has been successfully used by Hammerstein in the treatment of hirsutism (Hammerstein and Cupceancu 1969; Hammerstein et al. 1975). Hammerstein suggested the following therapeutic scheme: 500 µg ethinyl-oestradiol from the 5th to the 25th day of the menstrual cycle and 100 mg cyproterone acetate from the 5th to the 14th day only. This scheme was called "inversed sequential" and was possible because cyproterone acetate accumulates in fatty tissue and remains active up to 8 days after administration. The association with ethinyl-oestradiol ensures regular bleeding, reinforces the antigonadotropic effect of cyproterone acetate and therefore provides sure contraception. Nevertheless, its contra-indications remain the same as for synthetic oestrogens.

b) Personal Results

In a recent study (Kuttenn et al. 1980b), cyproterone acetate was associated with percutaneously administered natural 17β-oestradiol, which has none of the metabolic side effects of orally administered synthetic oestrogens. Twenty hirsute women, selected on the basis of their contra-indications to synthetic oestrogens (i.e. obesity, diabetes, hyperlipidaemia, hypertension), were studied. In nine cases, hirsutism was due to polycystic ovary syndrome. In 11 cases hirsutism was considered idiopathic.

The 20 patients have been treated for periods of 3–20 months and are still under treatment. Cyproterone acetate (50 mg) was administered daily from the 5th to the 25th day of the cycle. Oestradiol dissolved in an alcoholic excipient was applied to abdominal skin. Skin penetration was around 10% (Feldman and Maibach 1969), and menstruation ensued within 3 to 6 days after discontinuation of treatment.

The patients were clinically and biologically examined every 3 months. Hirsutism was estimated according to the classification of Ferriman and Gallway (1961). Moreover, as Ferriman does not take seborrhoea and acne into account, they were therefore evaluated on the basis of Cromencini's criteria (1976). The sum of these two estimations was used as the basic reference score in order to follow clinical evolution. Plasma testosterone, androstenedione, oestradiol, FSH and LH were assayed on the 15th day of the cycle. An additional plasma sample was taken on the 24th day of the same cycle for the assay of progesterone and oestradiol.

Clinical results proved surprisingly good. The initial mean clinical score for hirsutism plus seborrhoea and acne was 23.9 ± 5.1 for the 20 patients, with no significant difference between hirsutism of ovarian or idiopathic origin. This mean clinical score is represented as 100% in Fig 30. After 3 months, it was 65% of the original score, 48% after 6 months, 37% after 9 months and dropped to 22% after 12 months' treatment. Figure 30 also details the proportions of body and facial hair and seborrhoea and acne in the initial and subsequent scores: seborrhoea and acne decreased dramatically within the 1 month of treatment and practically disappeared

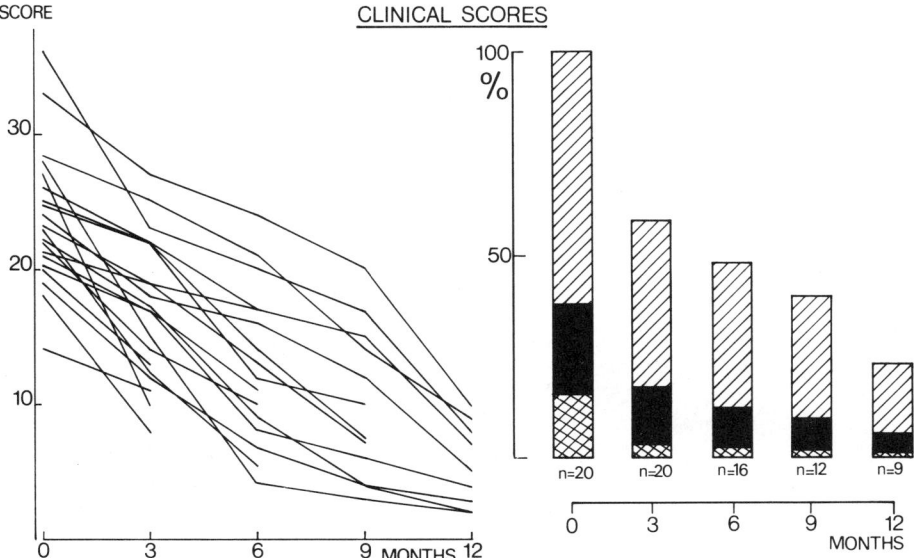

Fig. 30. Evolution of the clinical score of 20 hirsute women treated with oral cyproterone acetate and percutaneous oestradiol. On the *left*, individual values; on the *right*, the mean of the original scores is referred to as 100%. The percentage shown at 3, 6, 9 and 12 months treatment represents the mean percentage of each individual score. The respective proportions of body hair (▨), facial hair (■), acne and seborrhoea (▩) are represented in the initial and subsequent scores. Kuttenn et al. 1980b

after 3 months of treatment, whereas improvement in hirsutism appeared mainly after the 3rd month. Facial and body hair continuously improved to the same degree. By the end of 9 months' treatment, all the patients declared "being transformed". The patients who had been treated for 20 months no longer needed epilation.

Biologically, after 3 months' treatment, there was a significant ($P<0.001$) decrease in plasma testosterone and androstenedione from 64 ± 24 and 251 ± 100 ng/dl, respectively, to 25 ± 12 and 62 ± 21 ng/dl. Thereafter, plasma testosterone and androstenedione continued to decrease and, by the 9th month of treatment, they were respectively 21% and 11% of original values (Figs. 31, 32). Plasma androgen levels under treatment were not significantly different in the two groups of ovarian and idiopathic hirsutism.

Thus, a quick and clear clinical improvement occurred in the 20 patients. It should be noted that such a dramatic amelioration in such a short time is only possible by combining hormonal and aesthetic treatment. Electric epilation removes the old hair and cyproterone acetate prevents or slows down new hair growth. But this improvement contrasts with the mere stabilization obtained with oestrogen-progestogen association. In addition, it was observed to the same degree in all the cases of hirsutism, regardless of whether their origin was ovarian or idiopathic. This supports of the two levels of action of cyproterone acetate: suppression of androgen ovarian secretion and peripheral anti-androgen effect. A dose of 50 mg/day in adults is theoreticall insufficient to be antigonadotropic, but

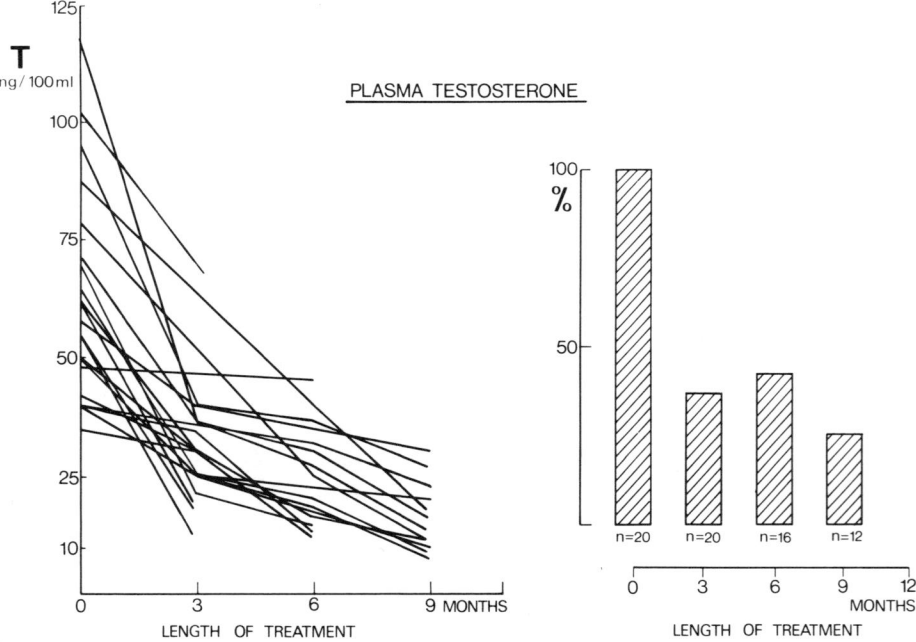

Fig. 31. Evolution of plasma testosterone (T) levels in 20 hirsute women treated with cyproterone acetate and percutaneous oestradiol. On the *left*, individual values; on the *right*, overall evolution expressed as the mean percentage of each individual plasma T level, the original score being 100%. Kuttenn et al. 1980b

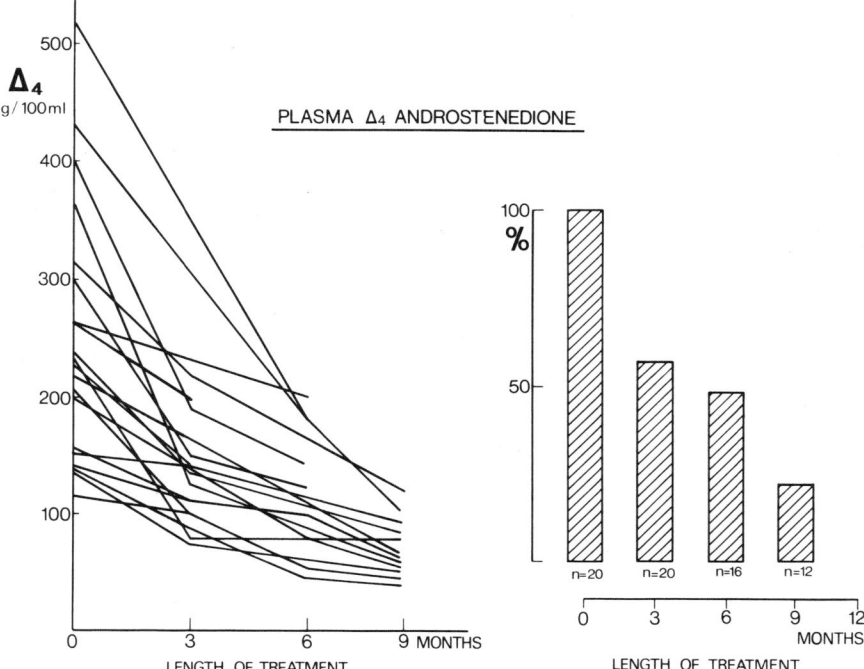

Fig. 32. Evolution of plasma androstenedione (Δ_4) levels in 20 hirsute women treated with cyproterone acetate and percutaneous oestradiol. On the *left*, individual values; on the *right*, overall evolution expressed as the mean percentage of each individual plasma Δ_4 level, the original score being 100%. Kuttenn et al. 1980b

after three treated cycles, a genuinely antigonadotropic effect is shown by dramatic decreases in plasma testosterone, androstenedione, oestradiol and LH and by the constant absence of plasma progesterone.

Plasma oestradiol levels dramatically fell under cyproterone acetate. It was 140 ± 62 pg/ml on the 24th day of the cycle before the treatment, it decreased to 48 ± 16 and 33 ± 10 pg/ml after 3 and 6 months' treatment with cyproterone acetate administration alone (15th day of the cycle). In the second period of treatment, when cyproterone acetate was associated with percutaneously administered oestradiol, plasma oestradiol levels ranged from 72 to 124 pg/ml. The administration of cyproterone acetate significantly decreased the levels of plasma LH from 4.0 ± 2.0 to 0.7 ± 0.4 mIU/ml ($P < 0.001$). As for plasma FSH, the tendency was not significant. The clinical improvement continued after testosterone and androstenedione levels became relatively stable, which can be considered as additional evidence of cyproterone acetate's peripheral effect.

In such an association, cyproterone acetate has a contraceptive effect due to its antigonadotropic action as well as to its luteomimetic activity which induces coagulation of the cervical mucus and atrophy of the endometrium. Percutaneously administered oestradiol is not used for its antigonadotropic effect, which is low at this dosage (Sitruk-Ware et al. 1980). Percutaneous oestradiol is essentially used as a substitutive therapy in order to provide physiological oestrogen levels necessary to maintain target organs' eutrophia. It also permits regular bleeding. The accumulation of cyproterone acetate in adipose tissue and its progressive release after treatment are probably responsible for prolonged progestative action and sometimes the absence or lateness of deprivation bleeding, despite discontinued administration of oestradiol.

As regards cyproterone acetate side effects, asthenia is one of the most common reported in the literature (Braendle et al. 1974; Hammerstein et al. 1975; Dewurst et al. 1977). It was long interpreted as a central sedative effect, or the result of cyproterone acetate slowing adrenal function (Zieger et al. 1976; Girard et al. 1978; Panesar and Stitch 1976). However, such side effects depended on the dose and duration of treatment. (Braendle et al. 1974; Jeffcoate et al. 1976). None of the patients treated by cyproterone acetate in combination with oestradiol, administered percutaneously, complained of asthenia. No hypotension or serum electrolyte abnormalities were noted. Plasma and urinary cortisol remained normal. No sign of adrenal insufficiency was observed by authors using 100 mg cyproterone acetate. The 50 mg dose is an even better guarantee in this respect.

Percutaneously administered oestradiol was preferred to oral synthetic oestrogens, usually combined with cyproterone acetate for its innocuity. (Ismail et al. 1974) Considerable evidence has become available concerning the harmful side effects of synthetic oestrogens (Cain et al. 1971; Beck 1973; Stern et al. 1976). Their toxicity depends on the distribution and the structure of the molecules. Oral administration concentrates oestrogens in the portal system and then increases their hepatic effects (Eisenfeld et al. 1978; Humpel et al. 1979). The oestrogen molecules with an ethinyl group at C 17 resist hepatic inactivation and therefore are most active on the hepatic receptors (Bolt et al. 1974; Valette et al. 1978). Hepatic toxicity is responsible for most of the side effects of sythetic oestrogens, i.e. hypertension, hyperlipidaemia, or alteration of coagulation factors.

Reducing the dosage does not avoid these side effects. Conjugated oestrogens per os have the same metabolic effects as sythetic oestrogens, since oral administration transforms the liver into a special target cell with predominant metabolism of oestradiol to oestrone, the hepatic impact of which is elevated.

"Natural" oestradiol, when administered by a route other than oral, has none of these deleterious effects (de Lignières and Mauvais-Jarvis 1976; Loeper et al. 1977; Steg et al. 1979; Basdevant and de Lignières 1980; Bercovici and Darragon 1980). Indeed, percutaneously applied oestrogen therapy appears quite beneficial since the natural oestradiol molecule can be used and the oestradiol/oestrone ratio is unaltered. In addition, it is possible to adjust plasma oestradiol levels (Sitruk-Ware et al. 1980).

The administration of cyproterone acetate in moderate sequential doses therefore provides considerable efficiency without the classic side effects. Its association with percutaneously administered oestradiol is another guarantee of metabolic safety. The rapid and dramatic improvement in hirsutism makes this therapy a method of choice in the treatment not only of hirsute women with contra-indications to synthetic oestrogens, but also in other cases of hirsutism, especially idiopathic hirsutism, in which cyproterone acetate could act directly on skin cytosolic receptors.

4. Corticosteroids

It is quite surprising to note that corticosteroids continue to be administered even though they are not expected to act by either blocking ovarian androgen secretion or by instituting peripheral androgen action. This type of treatment appears to be based on "old wives tales" and was given until recently, since there were few other therapeutic possibilities!

Corticosteroid treatment of hirsutism has also benefited from the belief that most cases of hirsutism were due to adrenal androgen overproduction. However, it has now been established: (1) that hirsutism due to adrenal overproduction, such as tumour/or enzymatic defect is rare, and (2) that the most frequent cases of hirsutism are either of ovarian origin, in which corticosteroid therapy is not helpful, or of idiopathic origin. In the latter case, when androgen overproduction exists, it is mainly of ovarian origin (Kirschner et al. 1976b).

The side effects of long-term corticosteroid therapy (signs of iatrogenic Cushing's syndrome), in addition to its slight efficiency, are good reasons to abandon it. Indeed, it seems only to make body hair brittle and to make scalp hair scarce — a fine result!!!

Corticosteroid therapy is only justified in congenital adrenal hyperplasia, in which it inhibits overproduction of pituitary ACTH and of adrenal androgens. The natural hormone, hydrocortisone, is generally preferable to dexamethasone. The dose should be adjusted, based on normalizing the plasma androstenedione (see Sect. I.I.8).

III. Conclusion

To be effective, the therapeutic battle against hirsutism must be waged on two fronts: hormonal and aesthetic. Aesthetic treatment removes the old hair and hormonal treatment slows down or prevents new hair growth.

Shaving must be avoided in all cases. Aesthetic treatment consists mainly of electric epilation, but should not start until androgen overproduction and peripheral utilization have been inhibited following 2 or 3 months of hormonal treatment. Electric epilation should only be performed by experts; it is mainly indicated on the face and may be associated with bleaching and hair removal by wax or tweezers in other parts of the body.

References

Abraham GE (1974) Ovarian and adrenal contribution to peripheral androgens during the menstrual cycle. J Clin Endocrinol Metab 39:340–346

Abraham GE (1978) Bilan et traitement de l'hyperandrogénie. In: Scholler R (éd) Endocrinologie de l'ovaire. Sepe, Paris, p 419

Abraham GE, Buster JE (1976) Peripheral and ovarian steroids in ovarian hyperthecosis. Obstet Gynecol 47:581:586

Abraham GE, Chakmakjian ZH (1973) Serum steroid levels during the menstrual cycle in a bilaterally adrenalectomized woman. J Clin Endocrinol Metab 37:581–587

Adachi K, Takayasu S, Takashima I, Kano M, Kondo S (1970) Human hair follicles: metabolism and control mechanisms. J Soc Cosmet Chem 21:901–924

Adashi EY, Rosenwaks Z, Lee PA, Seegar-Jones G, Migeon CJ (1979) Endocrine features of an adrenal like tumor of the ovary. J Clin Endocrinol Metab 48:241–245

Aiman J, Nalick RH, Jacobs A, Porter JC, Edman CD, Vellios F, MacDonald PC (1978) The origin of androgen and estrogen in a virilized postmenopausal woman with bilateral benign cystic teratomas. Obstet Gynecol 49:695–704

Amrhein JA, Meyer WJ III, Jones HW Jr, Migeon CJ (1976) Androgen insensitivity in man: evidence for genetic heterogeneity. Proc Natl Acad Sci USA 73:891–894

Amrhein JA, Klingesmith GJ, Walsh PC, Mc Kusick VA, Migeon CJ (1977) Partial androgen insensitivity: the Reifenstein syndrome revisited. N Engl J Med 297: 350–356

Ances IG, Ganis FM (1968) Metabolism of testosterone by virilizing Krukenberg tumor of the ovary. Am J Obst Gynecol 100:1062–1070

Anderson DC (1976) The role of sex hormone binding globulin in health and disease. In: James VHT, Serio M, Giusti G (eds) The endocrine function of the human ovary. Academic Press, New York, p 141

Anderson KM, Liao S (1968) Selective rentention of dihydrotestosterone by prostatic nuclei. Nature 219:277–278

Andre CM, James VHT (1974) Plasma androgens in idiopathic hirsutism. Steroids 24:295–303

Anliker R, Rohr O, Mart M (1956) Testostérone isolée d'une tumeur surrénale virilisante. Helv Chim Acta 39:100–1106

Apert M (1910) Hirsutisme et projeria. Bull Soc Pediat 12:501–515

Axelrod LR, Goldzieher JW (1961) Enzymatic inadequacies in human polycystic ovaries. Arch Biochem Biophys 95:547–548

Baird DT (1976) Ovarian steroid secretion and metabolism in women. In: James VHT, Serio M, Giusti G (eds) The endocrine function of the human ovary. Academic Press, New York, p 125

Baird DT, Horton R, Longcope C, Tait JF (1969) Steroid dynamics under steady-state conditions. Recent Prog Horm Res 25:611–656

Barbarino A, Perrelli L, Menini E (1976) Localization of a virilizing adrenal carcinoma by 131 I-19-iodocholesterol scintigraphy. J Nucl Biol Med 20:172–175

Barberia J, Pages L, Horton R (1976) Measurement of androstanediol in plasma in a radioimmunoassay using celite column chromatography. Fertil Steril 27:1101–1104

Bardin CW, Lipsett MB (1967) Testosterone and androstenedione blood production rates in normal women and women with idiopathic hirsutism or polycystic ovaries. J Clin Invest 46:891–902

Bardin CW, Mahoudeau JA (1970) Dynamics of androgen metabolism in women with hirsutism. Ann Clin Res 2:251–262

Bardin CW, Lipsett MB, Edgcombs JH, Marshall JR (1967) Studies of testosterone metabolism in a patient with masculinization due to stromal hyperthecosis. N Engl J Med 277:399–402

Bardin CW, Lipsett MB, French A (1968) Testosterone and androstenedione production rates in patients with metastatic adrenal cortical carcinoma. J Clin Endocrinol Metab 28:215–220

References

Bardin CW, Bullock LP, Sherins RJ, Mowszowicz I, Blackburn WR (1973) Androgen metabolism and mechanism of action in male pseudohermaphroditism: a study of testicular feminization. Recent Prog Horm Res 29:65–105

Barnes ND, Atherden SM (1972) Diagnosis of congenital adrenal hyperplasia by measurement of plasma 17-hydroxyprogesterone. Arch Dis Child 47:62–65

Barraclough CA, Gorski RA (1961) Evidence that the hypothalamus is responsible for androgen induced sterility. Endocrinology 68:68–79

Bartter FC, Henkin RI, Bryan GT (1968) Aldosterone hypersecretion in "non-salt-losing" congenital adrenal hyperplasia. J Clin Invest 47:1742–1752

Basdevant A, de Lignieres B (1980) Treatment of menopause by percutaneous administration of estradiol. In: Mauvais-Jarvis P, Vickers CFH, Wepierre J (eds) Percutaneous absorption of steroids. Academic Press, London, p 249–258

Baulieu EE (1962) Studies of conjugated 17-ketosteroids in a case of adrenal tumor. J Clin Endocrinol Metab 22:501–510

Baulieu EE, Jung I (1970) A prostatic cytosol receptor. Biochem Biophys Res Commun 38:599–606

Baulieu EE, Mauvais-Jarvis P (1964) Studies on testosterone metabolism. II Metabolism of testosterone-4-^{14}C and androst-4-ene-3, 17-dione-1, 2 ^{3}H. J Biol Chem 239:1578–1584

Baulieu EE, Peillon F, Migeon CJ (1967) Adrogenital syndrome. In: Einsenstein AB (ed) The adrenal cortex. Churchill, London, p 553

Baulieu EE, Lasnitzki I, Robel P (1968) Metabolism of testosterone and action of metabolites on prostate glands grown in organ culture. Nature 219:1155–1156

Beck P (1973) Contraceptive steroids: modifications of carbohydrate and lipid metabolism. Metabolism 22:841–852

Becker D, Schumacher P (1975) OP'DDD therapy in invasive adrenocortical carcinoma. Ann Intern Med 82:677–679

Bercovici JP, Darragon Th (1980) Les voies d'administration des stéroides sexuels naturels (estradiol, progestérone, testostérone). Nouv Presse Med 9:179–183

Bergenstal DM, Hertz R, Lipsett MB, Moy RH (1960) Chemotherapy of adrenocortical cancer with OP'DDD. Ann Int Med 53:672–682

Berger MJ, Taymor ML, Patton WC (1975) Gonadotropin levels and secretory patterns in patients with typical and atypical polycystic ovarian disease. Fertil Steril 26:619–626

Berliner DL, Pasqualini JR, Gallegos AJ (1968) The formation of water soluble steroids by human skin. J Invest Dermatol 50:220–224

Bingham KD, Shaw DA (1973) Male pattern baldness and the metabolism of androgens by human scalp skin. J Soc Cosmet Chem 24:523–536

Bird CE, Choong A, Knight L, Clark AF (1974) Kinetics of 5α-androstan-3α, 17β-diol metabolism in normal men and women. J Clin Endocrinol Metab 38:372–375

Birke G, Diczfaluzy E, Plantin LO, Robbe H, Westman A (1958) Familial congenital hyperplasia of the adrenal cortex. Acta Endocrinol (Copenh) 29:55–69

Birnholz JC (1973) Ultrasound imaging of adrenal mass lesions. Radiology 109:163–166

Blaquier J, Forchielli E, Dorfman RI (1967) In vitro metabolism of androgens in whole human blood. Acta Endocrinol (Copenh) 55:697–704

Blichert-Toft M, Vejlsted H, Kehlet H, Albrechtsen R (1975) Virilizing adrenocortical adenoma responsive to gonadotrophin. Acta Endocrinol (Copenh) 78:77–85

Blondeau JP, Corpechot C, Le Goascogne C, Baulieu EE, Robel P (1975) Androgen receptors in the rat ventral prostate and their hormonal control. Vitam Horm 33:319–345

Bolt HA, Kappus H, Kasbohrer R (1974) Metabolism of 17α-ethinylestradiol by human liver microsomes in vitro: aromatic hydroxylation and irreversible protein binding of metabolites. J Clin Endocrinol Metab 39:1072–1079

Bonaventura LM, Judd H, Roth LM, Clearly RE (1978) Androgen, estrogen and progestagen production by a lipid cell tumor of the ovary. Am J Obstet Gynecol 131:403–409

Bongiovanni AM, Eberlein WR (1958) Defective steroidal biogenesis in congenital adrenal hyperplasia. Pediatrics 21:661–672

Bongiovanni AM, Root AW (1963) The adrenogenital syndrome. N Engl J Med 268:1283–1289, 1342–1351

Bongiovanni AM, Eberlein WR, Goldmann AS, New M (1967) Disorders of adrenal steroid biogenesis. Rec Progr Horm Res 23:375–449

Bonne C, Saurat JH, Chivot M, Lehuchet D, Raynaud JP (1977) Androgen receptor in human skin. Brit J Dermatol 97:501–503

Bouchard PH, Kuttenn F, Mowszowicz I, Schaison G, Raux-Evrin MC, Mauvais-Jarvis P (1981) Congenital adrenal hyperplasia due to partial 21 hydroxylase deficiency. A study of five cases. Acta Endocrinol (Copenh) 96:107–111

Braendle W, Boess H, Breckwoldt M, Leven C, Bettendorf G (1974) Wirkung und Nebenwirkung der Cyproteronacetatbehandlung. Arch Gynaecol 216:335–345

Braithwaite SS, Erkman-Balis B, Avila TD (1979) Postmenopausal virilization due to ovarian stromal hyperthecosis. J Clin Endocrinol Metab 46:295–300

Brautbar N, Rosier A, Landau H, Cohen I, Nelken D, Cohen T, Levine C, Sack J, Benderli A, Moses S, Leiberman E, Dupont B, Levine LS, New MI (1979) No linkage between HLA and congenital adrenal hyperplasia due to 11-hydroxylase deficiency. N Engl J Med 300:205–206

Bricaire H, Luton JP (1977) L'OP'DDD possède-t-il une action antimitotique? Reflexions a propos de son emploi dans le traitement des adénocarcinomes surrénaliens. Nouv Press Med 6:36–50

Brook CGD, Zachman M, Prader A, Murset G (1974) Experience with long term therapy in congenital adrenal hyperplasia. J Pediatr 85:12–19

Brooks RV, Mattingly D, Mills IH, Prunty FTG (1960) Postpubertal adrenal virilism with biochemical disturbance of congenital type of adrenal hyperplasia. Br Med J I:1294–1298

Bruchovsky N (1971) Comparison of the metabolites formed in rat prostate following the in vivo administration of seven natural androgens. Endocrinology 89:1212–1222

Bruchovsky N, Wilson JD (1968) The conversion of testosterone to 5α-androstan-17β ol-3-one by rat prostate in vivo and in vitro. J Biol Chem 243:2012–2021

Bryan GT, Kliman B, Bartter FC (1965) Impaired aldosterone production in "salt-losing" congenital adrenal hyperplasia. J Clin Invest 44:957–965

Burger HG, Kent JR, Kellie AE (1964) Determination of testosterone in human peripheral and adrenal venous plasma. J Clin Endocrinol Metab 24:432–441

Burke CW, Anderson DC (1972) Sex hormone binding globulin is an estrogen amplifier. Nature 240:38–40

Burton RM, Westphal U (1972) Steroid hormone-binding proteins in blood plasma. Metabolism 21:253–276

Cain MD, Walters WA, Catt KJ (1971) Effects of oral contraceptive therapy on the renin angiotensin system. J Clin Endocrinol Metab 33:671–676

Calandra RS, Purvis K, Attramadal A, Hansson V (1977) Androgen receptors in the rat epididymis do not disappear after castration. J Steroid Biochem 8:1205–1206

Camacho AM, Migeon CJ (1963) Isolation, identification and quantitation of testosterone in the urine of normal adults and in patients with endocrine disorders. J Clin Endocrinol Metab 23:301–305

Camacho AM, Migeon CJ (1966) Testosterone excretion and production rate in normal adults and in patients with congenital adrenal hyperplasia. J Clin Endocrinol Metab 26:893–896

Cameron EH, Baillie AH, Grant JK, Milne JA, Thompson J (1966) Transformation in vitro of 7α-^{3}H-dehydroepiandrosterone to ^{3}H-testosterone by skin from men. J Endocrinol 35:XIX-XX

Casey JH, Nabarro JDN (1967) Plasma testosterone in idiopathic hirsutism, and the changes produced by adrenal and ovarian stimulation and suppression. J Clin Endocrinol Metab 27:1431–1435

Casey JH, Burger HG, Kent JR, Kellie AE, Moxham A, Nabarro J, Nabarro JDN (1966) Treatment of hirsutism by adrenal and ovarian suppression. J Clin Endocrinol Metab 26:1370–1374

Chen PS Jr, Mills IH, Bartter FC (1961) Ultrafiltration studies of steroid-protein binding. J Endocr 23:129–137

Cherif-Cheikh JL, de Lignieres B (1974) Traitment de la séborrhée du cuir chevelu par la progestérone percutanée. Sem Hop Ther 50:489–506

Childs B, Grumbach MM, Van Wyck JJ (1956) Virilizing adrenal hyperplasia: a genetic and hormonal study. J Clin Invest 35:213–222

Clark AF, Marcellus S, de Lory B, Bird CE (1975) Plasma testosterone free index: a better indicator of plasma androgen activity? Fertil Steril 26:1001–1011

Cleveland WW, Nikezic M, Migeon CJ (1962) Response to an 11β-hydroxylase inhibitor (SU-4885) in males with adrenal hyperplasia and their parents. J Clin Endocrinol Metab 22:281–286

Collier ME, Griffin JE, Wilson JD (1978) Intranuclear binding of ^{3}H-dihydrotestosterone by cultured human fibroblasts. Endocrinology 103:1499–1505

Coppage WS Jr, Cooner AE (1965) Testosterone in human plasma. N Engl J Med 273:902–907

References

Corvol PL, Bardin CW (1973) Species distribution of testosterone binding globulin. Biol Reprod 8:277–282

Corvol PL, Crambach A, Rodbard D, Bardin CW (1971) Physical properties and binding capacity of testosterone-estradiol binding globulin in human plasma determined by polyacrylamide gel electrophoresis. J Biol Chem 246:3435–3443

Cromencini C, Vignati E, Libroia A (1976) Treatment of hirsutism and acne in women with two combinations of cyproterone acetate and ethinyl estradiol. Acta Eur Fertil 7:299–314

Crooke AC, Butt WR, Paulmer R, Morris R, Edwards RL, Taylor CW, Short RV (1963) Effect of human pituitary follicle-stimulating hormone and chorionic gonadotropin in Stein-Leventhal syndrome. Br Med J I:1119–1123

Culiner A, Shippel S (1949) Virilism and theca-cell hyperplasia of the ovary syndrome. Br J Obstet Gynaecol 56:439–445

Danzo BJ, Eller BC, Orgebin-Crist MC (1974) Studies on the site of origin of the androgen binding protein present in epididymal cytosol from mature intact rabbits. Steroids 24:107–122

Decourt J, Jayle MF, Baulieu EE (1957) Virilisme cliniquement tardif avec excrétion de prégnanetriol et insuffisance de la production du cortisol. Ann Endocrinol (Paris) 18:416–422

Degenhart HJ, Visser HKA, Wilmink R, Croughs W (1965) Aldosterone and cortisol secretion rates in infants and children with congenital adrenal hyperplasia suggesting different 21-hydroxylation defects in salt-losers and non salt-losers. Acta Endocrinol (Copenh) 48:587–601

Dejong FH, Baird DT, Van Der Molen HJ (1974) Ovarian secretion rates of oestrogens androgens and progesterone in normal women and in women with persistent ovarian follicles. Acta Endocrinol (Copenh) 77:575–587

De Ligniéres B, Mauvais-Jarvis P (1976) Postmenopausal hormonal therapy. In: Scholler R (ed) Endocrinologie de l'ovaire. Sepe, Paris, p 541

De Moor P, Heyns W, Steeno O, Van Baelen H (1969) The steroid binding β-globulin in plasma: pathophysiological data. Ann Endocrinol [Suppl] 30:233–239

Dewurst CJ, Underhill R, Goldmann S, Mansfield M (1977) The treatment of hirsutism with cyproterone acetate (an antiandrogen). Br J Obstet Gynaecol 84:119–123

Dignam WJ, Pion RJ, Lamb EJ, Simmer HH (1964) Plasma androgens in women II Patients with polycystic ovaries and hirsutism. Acta Endocrinol (Copenh) 45:254–271

Dluhy RG, Barlow JJ, Mahoney EM, Shirley RL, Williams GH (1971) Profile and possible origin of an adrenocortical carcinoma. J Clin Endocrinol Metab 33:312–317

Dorfman RI (1967) The antiestrogenic and antiandrogenic activities of progesterone in the defense of normal fetus. Anat Rec 157: 547–557

Dorfman RI, Dorfman AS (1960) A test for antiandrogens. Acta Endocrinol (Copenh) 33:308–316

Dorfman RI, Forchielli E, Gut M (1963) Androgen biosynthesis and related studies. Recent Progr Horm Res 19:251–273

Dorfman RI, Shipley RA (1956) Androgens. Wiley & Sons, New York, p 116

Dorrington JH, Moon YS, Armstrong DT (1975) Estradiol-17β biosynthesis in cultured granulosa cells from hypophysectomized immature rats: stimulation by follicle stimulating hormone. Endocrinology 97:1328–1331

Dray F (1969) Physiopathologie de la liaison de la testostérone de l'estradiol et du cortisol aux protéines serigues. In: Rapports de la X° réunion des Endocrinologistes de Langue Française. Masson, Paris, p 159

Dray F, Sebaoun J, Mowszowicz I, Delzant G, Desgrez P, Gilbert-Dreyfus (1967) Facteurs influencant les taux de la testostérone plasmatique chez l'homme: rôle des hormones thyroidiennes. C R Acad Sci [D] (Paris) 264:2578–2579

Dray F, Sebaoun J, Delzant G, Ledru MJ, Mowszowicz I (1968 a) Activité de liaison de la testostérone dans le sérum des femmes présentant un virilisme pilaire idiopathique. Rev Franc Et Clin Biol 13:622–624

Dray F, Mowszowicz I, Ledru MJ, Sebaoun J, Delzant G, Crepy O, Schwob A (1968 b) La testostérone dans les thyrotoxycoses. In: Decourt J, Dreyfus G (eds) Actualités endocrinologiques. Expansion Scientifique, Paris, p 327

Ducharme JR, Forest MG, de Peretti E, Sempe M, Collu R, Bertrand J (1976) Plasma adrenal and gonadal sex steroids in human pubertal development. J Clin Endocrinol Metab 42:468–476

Dupont B, Oberfield EE, Smithwick EM, Lee TD, Levine LS (1977) Close genetic linkage between HLA and congenital adrenal hyperplasia (21-hydroxylase deficiency). Lancet 2:1309–1312

Eberlein WR, Bongiovani AM (1955) Congenital adrenal hyperplasia with hypertension: an unusual steroid pattern in blood and urine. J Clin Endocrinol Metab 15:1531–1534

Ebling FJ (1976) Hair. J Invest Dermatol 67:98–105

Ebling FJ, Ebling E, McCaffery V, Skinner J (1973) The responses of the sebaceous glands of the hypophysectomized castrated male rat to 5α-androstanedione and 5α-androstane-3β, 17β-diol. J Invest Dermatol 60:183–187

Echt CR, Hadd HE (1968) Androgen excretion patterns in a patient with a metastatic hilus cell tumor of the ovary. Am J Obstet Gynecol 100:1055–1070

Eisenfeld AJ, Ajew RF, Weinberger MH (1978) Oral contraceptives possible mediation of side effects via an estrogen receptor in liver. Biochem Pharmacol 27:2571–2575

Erickson GF, Hsueh AJW (1978) Stimulation of aromatase activity by follicle stimulating hormone in rat granulosa cells in vivo and in vitro. Endocrinology 102:1275–1282

Erickson GF, Hsueh AJW, Quigley ME, Rebar RW, Yen SSC (1979) Functional studies of aromatase activity in human granulosa cells from normal and polycystic ovaries. J Clin Endocrinol Metab 49:514–519

Evain D, Morera AM, Saez JM (1976) Glucocorticoid receptors in interstitial cells of the rat testis. J Steroid Biochem 7:1135–1140

Evain D, Savage MO, Binet E (1977) A specific and rapid determination of human skin dihydrotestosterone cytosol receptor. J Clin Endocrinol Metab 45:363–366

Fahmy D, Griffiths K, Turnbull AC, Symington T (1968) A comparison of the metabolism in vitro of 7-^{3}H-dehydroepiandrosterone sulfate and 4-C^{14} pregnenolone by tissue from a hilus cell tumor of the ovary. J Endocrinol 41:61–68

Fang S, Liao S (1969) Antagonistic action of antiandrogens on the formation of a specific dihydrotestosterone-receptor protein complex in rat ventral prostate. Mol Pharmacol 5:428–431

Faredin I, Fazekas AG, Kokai K, Toth I, Julesz M (1967) The in vitro metabolism of 4-^{14}C-dehydroepiandrosterone by human male pubic skin. Eur J Steroids 2:223–242

Feldman RJ, Maibach HI (1969) Percutaneous penetration of steroids in man. J Invest Dermatol 52:89–94

Ferriman D, Gallway JD (1961) Clinical assessment of body hair in women. J Clin Endocrinol Metab 24:1440–1448

Flamigni C, Collins WP, Koullapnis EN, Craft I, Dewhurst CJ, Sommerville IF (1971) Androgen metabolism in human skin. J Clin Endocrinol Metab 32:737–743

Fraenkel L (1943) Thecoma and hyperthecosis of the ovary. J Clin Endocrinol Metab 3:557–599

Franks RC (1974) Plasma 17-hydroxyprogesterone, 21-deoxycortisol and cortisol in congenital adrenal hyperplasia. J Clin Endocrinol Metab 39:1099–1102

Frederiksen DW, Wilson JD (1971) Partial characterization of the nuclear reduced adenine dinucleotide phosphate: Δ_4-3-ketosteroid-5α-oxydoreductase of rat prostate. J Biol Chem 246:2584–2593

Fukushima DK, Bradlow HL, Hellman L, Zumoff B, Gallagher TF (1961) Study of 17-hydroxyprogesterone-4-C^{14} in man. J Clin Endocrinol Metab 21:765–778

Fukushima DK, Finkelstein JW, Yoshida F, Boyar RM, Hellman L (1975) Pituitary adrenal activity in untreated congenital adrenal hyperplasia. J Clin Endocrinol Metab 40:1–12

Futterweit W, McNiven NL, Guena-Garcia R, Gibree N, Drosdowsky M, Siegel GL, Soffer LJ, Rosenthal IM, Dorfman RI (1964) Testosterone in human urine. Steroids 4:137–141

Futterweit W, Freeman R, Siegel GL, Griboff SI, Dorfmann RI, Soffer LJ (1965) Clinical application of a gas chromatographic method for the combined determination of testosterone and epitestosterone glucuronide in urine. J Clin Endocrinol Metab 25:1451–1456

Gabrilove JL, Sharma PC, Dorfman RI (1965) Adrenocortical 11β-hydroxylase deficiency and virilism first manifest in the adult woman. N Engl J Med 272:1189–1194

Gabrilove JL, Nicolis GL, Mitty HA (1976) Virilizing adrenocortical adenoma studied by selective adrenal venography. Am J Obstet Gynecol 125:180–184

Gallagher TF, Spencer H, Bradlow HL, Allen L, Hellman L (1962) Steroid production and metabolism in metastatic arrhenoblastoma. J Clin Endocrinol Metab 22:970–977

Gallais A (1912) Le syndrome surrénogenital. Thesis, University of Paris, Vigot, 1914

Gallegos AJ, Berliner DL (1967) Transformation and conjugation of dehydroepiandrosterone by human skin. J Clin Endocrinol Metab 27:1214–1218

Gambrell RD, Greenblatt RB, Mahesh VB (1973) Inappropriate secretion of LH in the Stein-Leventhal syndrome. Obstet Gynecol 42:429–440

Gandy HM, Peterson RE (1968) Measurement of testosterone and 17-ketosteroids in plasma by double isotopic dilution derivative technique. J Clin Endocrinol Metab 28:949–977

Garvin AJ, Pratt-Thomas HR, Spector M, Spicer SS, Williamson HO (1976) Gonadoblastoma: histologic ultrastructural and histochemical observations in five cases. Am J Obstet Gynecol 125:459–471

Giacomini M, Wright F (1980) The effects of progesterone and pregnanedione on the reductive metabolism of dihydrotestosterone in human skin. J Steroid Biochem 13:645–651

Gillette JR (1967) Individually different responses to drugs according to age, sex and functional or pathological state. In: Wolstenholme GEW, Porter R (eds) Ciba foundation on drug responses in man. Churchill, London, p 12

Girard J, Baumann JB, Buchler U, Zuppinger K, Haas HG, Staub JJ, Wyss HI (1978) Cyproterone acetate and ACTH adrenal function. J Clin Endocrinol Metab 47:581–586

Givens JR (1976) Hirsutism and hyperandrogenism. Adv Intern Med 21:221–247

Givens JR, Wiser WL, Coleman SA, Wilroy RS, Andersen RN, Fish SA (1971) Familial ovarian hyperthecosis: a study of two families. Am J Obstet Gynecol 110:959–972

Givens JR, Andersen RN, Wiser WL, Coleman SA, Fish SA (1974) A gonadotropin responsive adrenocortical adenoma. J Clin Endocrinol Metab 38:126–133

Givens JR, Andersen RN, Wiser WL, Umstot ES, Fish SA (1976a) The effectiveness of two oral contraceptives in suppressing plasma androstenedione, testosterone, LH and FSH, and in stimulating plasma testosterone binding capacity in hirsute women. Am J Obstet Gynecol 124:333–339

Givens JR, Andersen RN, Umstot ES, Wiser WL (1976b) Clinical findings and hormonal responses in patient with polycystic ovarian disease with normal versus elevated LH levels. Obstet Gynecol 47:388–394

Gomez EC, Hsia SL (1968) In vitro metabolism of testosterone-4-^{14}C and Δ_4-androstene-3, 17 dione 4-^{14}C in human skin. Biochemistry 7:24–32

Gomez EC, Hsia SL, Frost P (1972) Cutaneous transformation of testosterone into 5α-androstene-3β diol. J Clin Endocrinol Metab 34:417–419

Gordon GG, Southren AL, Tochimoto S, Rand JJ, Olivo J (1969) Effect of hyperthyroidism and hypothyroidism on the metabolism of testosterone and androstenedione in man. J Clin Endocrinol Metab 29:164–170

Gordon GG, Southren AL, Tochimoto S, Olivo J, Altman K, Rand J, Lemberger L (1970) Effect of medroxyprogesterone acetate (Provera) on the metabolism and biological activity of testosterone. J Clin Endocrinol Metab 30:449–456

Gourmelen M, Pham-Huu-Trung MT, Bredon MG, Girard F (1979) 17-hydroxyprogesterone in the cosyntropin test: results in normal and hirsute women and in mild congenital adrenal hyperplasia. Acta Endocrinol (Copenh) 90:481–489

Govan ADT, Woodcock AS, Gowing NFC, Langley FA, Neville AM, Anderson MC (1977) A clinico-pathological study of gonadoblastoma. Br J Obstet Gynaecol 84:222–228

Green OC, Migeon CJ, Wilkins L (1960) Urinary Steroids in hypertensive form of congenital adrenal hyperplasia. J Clin Endocrinol Metab 20:929–946

Greenblatt RB, Colle ML, Mahesh VB (1976) Ovarian and adrenal steroid production in the postmenopausal woman. Obstet Gynecol 47:383–387

Griffin JE, Wilson JD (1980) The syndrome of androgen resistance. N Engl J med 302:198–209

Griffin JE, Punyashthiti K, Wilson JD (1976) Dihydrotestosterone binding by cultured human fibroblasts. J Clin Invest 57:1342–1351

Grodin JM, Siiteri PK, MacDonald PC (1973) Source of estrogen production in postmenopausal women. J Clin Endocrinol Metab 36:207–214

Gueriguian JL, Pearlman WH (1968) Some properties of testosterone binding component of human pregnancy serum. J Biol Chem 243:5226–5233

Gutai JP, Kowarski AA, Migeon CJ (1977) The detection of the heterozygous carrier for congenital virilizing adrenal hyperplasia. Pediatrics 90:924–929

Habrioux G, Desfosses B, Condom R, Faure B, Jayle MF (1978) Simultaneous radioimmunoassay of 5α-androstane-3α, 17β-diol and 5α-androstane-3β, 17β-diol unconjugated and conjugated in human serum. Steroids 32:61–71

Hall R, Smith PA, Harkness RA, Smart GA (1970) A study of the parents of patients with congenital adrenal hyperplasia; detection of the heterozygote. Proc R Soc Med 63:1040–1042

Hamada H, Neumann F, Junkmann K (1963) Intrauterine antimaskuline Beeinflussung von Rattenfeten durch ein stark gestagen wirksames Steroid. Acta Endocrinol (Copenh) 44:380–388

Hammerstein J, Cupceancu B (1969) Behandlung des Hirsutismus durch Cyproterone Acetat. Dtsch Med Wochenschr 94:829–834

Hammerstein J, Meckies J, Leo-Rossberg I, Moltz L, Zielske F (1975) Use of cyproterone acetate (CPA) in the treatment of acne, hirsutism and virilism. J Steroid Biochem 6:827–836

Hamvi GS, Serbin RA, Kruger FA (1957) Does adrenocortical hyperplasia result in adrenocortical carcinoma? N Engl J Med 257:1153–1157

Harper ME, Pierrepoint CG, Fahmy AR, Griffiths K (1970) The effect of prostatic metabolites of testosterone and other substances on the isolated deoxyribonucleic acid polymerase of the canine prostate. Biochem J 119:785–786

Harrison JH, Mahoney EM, Bennett AH (1973) Tumors of the adrenal cortex. Cancer 32:1227–1235

Hopkinson CRN, Park BK, Johnson MW, Sturm G, Steinbach K, Kirchhauser C (1977) Concentrations of unconjugated 5α-androstan-3β, 17β-diol in human peripheral plasma as measured by radioimmunoassay. J Steroid Biochem 8:1253–1257

Horton R, Frasier SD (1967) Androstenedione and its conversion to plasma testosterone in congenital adrenal hyperplasia. J Clin Invest 46:1003–1009

Horton R, Neisler J (1968) Plasma androgens in patients with the polycystic syndrome. J Clin Endocrinol Metab 28:479–484

Horton R, Tait JF (1966) Androstenedione production and interconversion rates measured in peripheral blood and studies on the possible sites of its interconversion to testosterone. J Clin Invest 45:301–313

Horton R, Tait JF (1967) In vivo conversion of dehydroisoandrosterone to plasma androstenedione and testosterone in man. J Clin Endocrinol Metab 27:79–88

Hosseinian AH, Kim MH, Rosenfield RL (1976) Obesity and oligomenorrhea are associated with hyperandrogenism independant of hirsutism. J Clin Endocrinol Metab 42:765–769

Hughes IA, Winter JS (1976) The application of a serum 17-OH-progesterone radioimmunoassay to the diagnosis and management of congenital adrenal hyperplasia. J Pediatr 88:766–773

Humpel M, Nieuweboer B, Wendt H, Speck U (1979) Investigations of pharmacokinetics of ethinyl estradiol to specific consideration of a possible first pass effect in women. Contraception 19:421–431

Hutter AM, Kayhoe DE (1966 a) Adrenal cortical carcinoma: clinical features of 138 patients. Am J Med 41:572–580

Hutter AM, Kayhoe DE (1966 b) Adrenal cortical carcinoma. Results of treatment with OP'DDD in 138 patients. Am J Med 41:581–592

Huvos AG, Hadji SI, Brasfield RD (1970) Adrenal cortical carcinoma. Clinicopathological study of 34 cases. Cancer 25:354–361

Imperato-McGinley J, Guerrero L, Gautier T, Peterson RE (1974) Steroid 5α-reductase deficiency in man: an inherited form of male pseudohermaphroditism. Science 186:1213–1215

Ismail AAA, Loraine JA (1969) Hirsutism: a disorder frequently associated with menstrual abnormalities. Clin Obstet Gynecol 12:800–827

Ismail AAA, Davidson DW, Souka AP, Barnes EW, Irvine WJ, Kilimnik H, Wanderbeeken Y (1974) The evaluation of the role of androgens in hirsutism and the use of a new antiandrogen "cyproterone acetate" for therapy. J Clin Endocrinol Metab 39:81–95

Ito R, Horton R (1971) The source of plasma dihydrotestosterone in man. J Clin Invest 50:1621–1627

James VHT, Rippon AE, Jacobs HS (1976) Plasma androgens in patients with hirsutism. In: James VHT, Serio M, Giusti G (eds) The endocrine function of the human ovary. Academic Press, New York, p 457

Jayle MF, (1967) Exploration dynamique des fonctions endocrines de l'ovaire. In: Jayle MF (ed) Fonctions endocrines de l'ovaire. Gauthier-Villars, Paris, p 447

Jayle MF, Weinmann SH, Baulieu EE, Vallin Y (1958) Virilisme post pubertaire discret par déficience de l'hydroxylation en C_{21}. Acta Endocrinol (Copenh) 29:513–524

Jayle MF, Scholler R, Mauvais-Jarvis P, Szper M (1962) Exploration dynamique de la fonction ovarienne par les gonadotrophines chorioniques associées a la dexamethasone. Clin Chim Acta 7:322–328

Jeffcoate SL, Prunty FTG (1968) Steroid synthesis in vitro by a hilar cell tumor. Am J Obstet Gynecol 101:684–688

Jeffcoate WJ, Edwards CRW, Rees LH, Besser GM (1976) Cyproterone acetate. Lancet II:1190–1191

Jenkins JS, Ash S (1971) The metabolism of testosterone by skin in normal subjects and in testicular feminization. J Endocrinol 49:515–520

Jewelewicz R, Warren M, Dyrenfurth I, Vande Wiele RL (1971) Physiological studies with purified human pituitary FSH (HP-FSH). J Clin Endocrinol Metab 32:688–691

Jones HW JR, Jones GES (1954) The gynecological aspects of adrenal hyperplasia and allied disorders. Am J Obstet Gynecol 68:1330–1365

Jones GES, Howard JE, Langfort H (1953) The use of cortisone in follicular phase disturbances. Fertil Steril 4:49–62

Judd HL, Yen SSC (1973) Serum androstenedione and testosterone levels during the menstrual cycle. J Clin Endocrinol Metab 36:475–481

Judd JL, Scully RE, Herbst AL, Yen SSC, Ingersol FM, Kliman B (1973) Familial hyperthecosis: comparison of endocrinologic and histologic findings with polycystic ovarian disease. Am J Obstet Gynecol 117:976–982

Judd HL, Judd GE, Lucas WE, Yen SSC (1974) Endocrine function of the post menopausal ovary: concentration of androgens and estrogens in ovarian and peripheral vein blood. J Clin Endocrinol Metab 39:1020–1023

Juneja HS, Motta M, Vasconi F, Martini L (1977) Negative and positive effects of androgens on gonadotropin release. In: Martini L, Motta M (eds) Androgens and antiandrogens. Raven, New York, p 127

Kapler E, Sprague E, Mason H, Power M (1948) The pathologic physiology of adrenal cortical tumors and Cushing's syndrome. Recent Progr Horm Res 2:345–364

Karam K, Hajj S (1979) Hyperthecosis syndrome. Acta Obstet Gynecol Scand 58:73–79

Kase N, Conrad SH (1964) Steroid biosynthesis in abnormal ovaries. I Arrhenoblastoma. Am J Obstet Gynecol 90:1251–1261

Kato T, Horton R (1968) Studies of testosterone binding globulin. J Clin Endocrinol Metab 28:1160–1168

Kaufman M, Pinsky L, Straisfeld C, Shanfield B, Zilahi B (1975) Qualitative differences in testosterone metabolism as an indication of cellular heterogeneity in fibroblasts monolayers derived from human preputial skin. Exp Cell Res 96:31–36

Kaufman M, Straisfeld C, Pinsky L (1976) Male pseudohermaphroditism presumably due to target organ unresponsiveness to androgens. Deficient 5α-dihydrotestosterone binding in cultured skin fibroblasts. J Clin Invest 58:345–350

Keenan BS, Meyer WJ III, Hadjian AJ, Jones HW, Migeon CJ (1974) Syndrome of androgen insensitivity in man: absence of 5α-dihydrotestosterone binding in skin fibroblasts. J Clin Endocrinol Metab 38:1143–1146

Keenan BS, Meyer WJ III, Hadjian AJ, Migeon CT (1975) Androgen receptor in human skin fibroblasts: characterization of a specific 17β-hydroxy-5α-androstan-3-one protein complex in cell sonicates and nuclei. Steroids 25:535–552

Kennedy BJ, Nathanson IT (1953) Effect of intensive sex steroid hormone therapy in advanced breast cancer. JAMA 152:1135–1141

Kerkay J, Westphall U (1968) Steroid-protein interactions. XIX. Complex formation between α1-acid glycoprotein and steroid hormones. Biochem Biophys Acta 170:324–333

Kinouchi T, Horton R (1974) 3α-androstanediols kinetics in man. J Clin Invest 54:646–653

Kirschner MA, Bardin CW (1972) Androgen production and metabolism in normal and virilized women. Metabolism 21:667–688

Kirschner MA, Jacobs JB (1971) Combined ovarian and adrenal vein catheterization to determine the site(s) of androgen overproduction in hirsute women. J Clin Endocrinol Metab 33:199–207

Kirschner MA, Sinhamahapatra S, Zucker IR, Loriaux L, Nieschlag E (1973) The production origin and role of dehydroepiandrosterone and Δ_5-androstenediol as androgen prehormones in hirsute women. J Clin Endocrinol Metab 37:183–189

Kirschner MA, Zucker IR, Jespersen DL (1976 a) Ovarian and adrenal vein catheterization studies in women with idiopathic hirsutism. In: James VHT, Serio M, Giusti G (eds) The endocrine function of the human ovary. Academic Press, New York, p 443

Kirschner MA, Zucker IR, Jesperson D (1976 b) Idiopathic hirsutism an ovarian abnormality. N Engl J Med 294:637–640

Knorr D, Bidlingmaier F, Butenandt O, von Schnakenburg K, Wagner W (1975) A test for heterozygosity in congenital adrenal hyperplasia (abstr 6). Pediatr. Res 9:681

Knorr D, Bidlingmaier F, Butenandt O, Von Schnakenburg K, Wagner W (1977) Test for heterozigosity of congenital adrenal hyperplasia. In: Lee PA, Platnick L, Kowarski A, Migeon CJ (eds) Congenital adrenal hyperplasia. University Park Press, Baltimore, p 495

Korenman SG, Lipsett MB (1964) Is testosterone glucuronide uniquely derived from plasma testosterone? J Clin Invest 43:2125–2133

Korenman SG, Wilson H, Lipsett MB (1963) Testosterone production rates in normal adults. J Clin Invest 42:1753–1762

Korenman SG, Kirshner MA, Lipsett MB (1965) Testosterone production in normal, virilized women and in women with the Stein-Leventhal syndrome or idiopathic hirsutism. J Clin Endocrinol Metab 25:798–803

Korth-Schutz S, Levine LS, Roth JA, Saenger P, New MI (1977) Virilizing adrenal tumor in a child suppressed with dexamethasone for three years. Effect of OP'DDD on serum and urinary androgens. J Clin Endocrinol Metab 44:433–439

Korth-Schutz S, Virdis R, Saenger P, Chow DR, Levine LS, New MI (1978) Serum androgens as a continuing index of adequacy of treatment of congenital adrenal hyperplasia. J Clin Endocrinol Metab 46:452–458

Kowarski A, Finkelstein JS, Spaulding JS, Holman GH, Migeon CJ (1965) Aldosterone secretion rate in congenital adrenal hyperplasia. J Clin Invest 44:1505–1513

Krensky AM, Bongiovanni AM, Marino I, Parks I, Tenore A (1977) Identification of heterozygote carriers of congenital adrenal hyperplasia by radioimmunoassay of serum 17-OH progesterone. J pediatr 90:930–933

Krieg M, Smith K, Bartsch W (1978) Demonstration of a specific androgen receptor in heart muscle: relationship between binding, metabolism and tissue levels of androgens. J Clin Endocrinol Metab 103:1686–1694

Kulin HE, Reiter EO (1976) Gonadotropin and testosterone measurement after estrogen administration to adult men, prepubertal and puberal boys and men with hypogonadotropism: evidence for maturation of positive feedback in the male. Pediatr Res 10:46–51

Kuttenn F, Mauvais-Jarvis P (1975) Testosterone 5α-reduction in the skin of normal subjects and of patients with abnormal sex development. Acta Endocrinol (Copenh) 79:164–176

Kuttenn F, Mauvais-Jarvis P (1978) L'hirsutisme. J Gynecol Obstet Biol Reprod (Paris) 7:693–701

Kuttenn F, Mowszowicz I, Schaison G, Mauvais-Jarvis P (1977) Androgen production and skin metabolism in hirsutism. J Endocrinol 75:83–91

Kuttenn F, Wright F, Mowszowicz I, Baudot N, Giacomini M, Mauvais-Jarvis P (1979 a) Physiologie du récepteur cutané humain. In: Les androgènes. Masson, Paris, p 65

Kuttenn F, Mowszowicz I, Wright F, Baudot N, Jaffiol C, Robin M, Mauvais-Jarvis P (1979 b) Male pseudohermaphroditism: a comparative study of one patient with 5α-reductase deficiency and three patients with the complete form of testicular feminization. J Clin Endocrinol Metab 49:861–865

Kuttenn F, Mowszowicz I, Mauvais-Jarvis P (1980 a) Androgen metabolism in human skin. In: Mauvais-Jarvis P, Vickers CFH, Wepierre J (eds) Percutaneous absorption of steroids. Academic Press London, p 99

Kuttenn F, Rigaud C, Wright F, Mauvais-Jarvis P (1980 b) Treatment of hirsutism by oral cyproterone acetate and percutaneous oestradiol. J Clin Endocrinol Metab 51:1107–1111

Laband P, Tresguerres JAF, Lisboa BP, Volkwein U, Tamm J (1978) The determination of 5α-androstane-3α, 17β-diol in human plasma by radioimmunoassay. Acta Endocrinol (Copenh) 88:778–786

Laffargue P, Payan H, Rampal M, Coignet J, Piana L (1968) Lutéome sécrétant ou hyperplasie stromale lutéinisée de l'ovaire gravide. Presse Méd 76:155–158

Lamberigts G, Dierickx P, DeMoor P, Verhoeven G (1979) Comparison of the metabolism and receptor binding of testosterone and 17β-hydroxy-5α-androstan-3-one in normal skin fibroblasts cultures: influence of origin and passage number. J Clin Endocrinol Metab 49:924–930

Laschet U, Laschet L, Fetzner HR, Glaesel HU, Mall G, Naab M (1967) Results in the treatment of hyper or abnormal sexuality of men with antiandrogens. (Abstr 38) Acta Endocrinol [Suppl] (Copenh) 119:54

Lasnitzki I, Franklin HR (1975) The influence of serum on uptake, conversion and action of testosterone in rat prostate glands in organ culture. J Endocrinol 64:289–297

Lee PA, Gareis FJ (1975) Evidence for partial 21-hydroxylase deficiency among heterozygote carriers of congenital adrenal hyperplasia. J Clin Endocrinol Metab 41:415–418

Leichter SB, Jacobs LS (1976) Normal gestation and diminished androgen responsiveness in an untreated patient with 21-hydroxylase deficiency. J Clin Endocrinol Metab 42:575–581

Lerner LJ (1964) Hormone antagonists: inhibition of specific activities of estrogen and androgen. Recent Prog Horm Res 20:435–476

Leshin M, Griffin JE, Wilson JD (1978) Hereditary male pseudohermaphroditism associated with an unstable form of 5α-reductase. J Clin Invest 62:685–691

Levine LS, Rauh W, Gottesdiener K, Chow D, Gunczler P, Rappaport R, Pang S, Schneider B, New MI (1980). New studies of the 11β-hydroxylase and 18-hydroxylase enzymes in the hypertensive form of congenital adrenal hyperplasia. J Clin Endocrinol Metab 50:258–263

Liao S (1977) Molecular actions of androgens. In: Litwack C (ed) BiochemicaL actions of steroid hormones. Academic Press New York, p 351

Liddle GW (1960) Tests of pituitary-adrenal suppressibility in diagnosis of Cushing's syndrome. J Clin Endocrinol Metab 20:1559–1560

Lippe BM, La Franchi SH, Lavin N, Parlow A, Coyotupa J, Kaplan SA (1974) Serum 17α-hydroxyprogesterone, progesterone, estradiol and testosterone in the diagnosis and management of congenital adrenal hyperplasia. J Pediatrics 85:782–787

Lipsett MB, Wilson HM (1962) Adrenocortical cancer: steroid biosynthesis and metabolism evaluated by urinary metabolites. J Clin Endocrinol Metab 22:906–915

Lipsett MB, Hertz R, Ross GT (1963) Chemical and pathophysiologic aspects of adrenocortical carcinoma. Am J Med 35:374–383

Lipsett MB, Kirschner MA, Wilson H, Bardin CW (1970) Malignant lipid cell tumor of the ovary. Clinical, biochemical and etiologic considerations. J Clin Endocrinol Metab 30:336–344

Lloyd CW (1966) Androgen in the female. Trans New Engl Obstet Gynecol Soc 20:53–65

Lloyd CW, Lobotsky J, Segre EJ, Kobayashi T, Taymor ML, Batt RE (1966) Plasma testosterone and urinary 17-ketosteroids in women with idiopathic hirsutism and polycystic ovaries. J Clin Endocrinol Metab 26:314–324

Loeper J, Loeper J, Ohlghiesser C, de Ligniéres B, Mauvais-Jarvis P (1977) Influence de l'estrogénothérapie sur les triglycérides. Nouv Presse Med 6:2747–2750

Loriaux DL, Ruder HJ, Lipsett MB (1974) Plasma steroids in congenital adrenal hyperplasia. J Clin Endocrinol Metab 39:627–630

Lubicz-Nawrocki CM (1973) The effects of metabolites of testosterone on the viability of hamster epididymal spermatozoa. J Endocrinol 58:193–198

Lubitz JA, Freeman L, Okun R (1973) Mitotane use in inoperable adrenal cortical carcinoma. JAMA 223:1109–1112

Maes M, Sultan C, Zerhouni N, Rothwell SW, Migeon CJ (1979) Role of testosterone binding to the androgen receptor in male sexual differenciation of patients with 5α-reductase deficiency. J Steroid Biochem 11:1385–1390

Mahesh VB, Greenblatt RB (1964) Steroid secretion of the normal and polycystic ovary. Rec Prog Horm Res 20:392

Mahesh VB, Greenblatt RB, Aydar CK, Roy S, Puebla RA, Ellegood JO (1964) Urinary steroid excretion patterns in hirsutism. I. use of adrenal and ovarian suppression tests in the study of hirsutism. J Clin Endocrinol Metab 24:1283–1292

Mahesh VB, Greenblatt RB, Coniff RF (1968) Urinary steroid excretion before and after dexamethasone administration and steroid content of adrenal tissue and venous blood in virilizing adrenal tumors. Am J Obstet Gynecol 100:1043–1054

Mahesh VB, McDonough PG, Deleo CA (1970) Endocrine studies in the arrhenoblastoma. Am J Obst Gynecol 107:183–187

Mahoudeau JA, Corvol P (1973) Rabbit testosterone binding globulin. I Physicochemical properties. Endocrinology 92:1113–1119

Mahoudeau JA, Bardin CW, Lipsett MB (1971) The metabolic clearance rate and origin of plasma dihydrotestosterone in man and its conversion to the 5α-androstanediols. J Clin Invest 50:1338–1344

Mainwaring WIP (1977) The mechanism of action of androgens. Springer, Berlin Heidelberg New York

Mainwaring WIP, Irving Ra (1973) The use of deoxyribose-nucleic and cellulose chromatography and isoelectro-focusing for the characterization and partial purification of steroid-receptor complexes. Biochem J 134:113–127

Mangan FR, Mainwaring WIP (1972) An explanation of the antiandrogenic properties of 6α-bromo-17β-hydroxy-17α-methyl-4-oxa-5α-androstane-3-one. Steroids 20:331–343

Mangan FR, Neal GE, Williams DC (1967) The effects of diethylstilboestrol and castration on the nucleic acid and protein metabolism of rat prostate gland. Biochem J 104:1075–1081

Mansuwan K, Kalant N (1965) Urinary excretion of testosterone in idiopathic hirsutism. Proc Soc Exp Biol Med 119:911–918

Maroulis GB, Abraham GE (1976) Ovarian and adrenal contributions to peripheral steroid levels in postmenopausal women. Obstet Gynecol 48:150–154

Maroulis GB, Manlimos FS, Abraham GE (1977) Comparison between urinary 17-ketosteroids and serum androgens in hirsute patients. Obstet Gynecol 49:454–458

Marsh JM, Savard IC, Lemaire WJ (1976) Steroidogenic capacities of the different compartments of the human ovary In: James VHT, Serio M, Giusti G (eds) The endocrine function of human ovary. Academic Press, New York, p 37

Massa R, Martini L (1971) Interference with the 5α-reductase system. A new approach for developping antiandrogens. Gynec Invest 2:253–270

Mauthe I, Laspe H, Knorr D (1977) Zur Häufigkeit des kongenitalen adrenogenitalen Syndroms (AGS): München 1963–1972. Klin Paediatr 189:172–176

Mauvais-Jarvis P (1977) Androgen metabolism in human skin: mechanisms of control. In: Martini L, Motta M (eds) Androgens and antiandrogens. Raven, New York, p 229

Mauvais-Jarvis P, Kuttenn F (1973) L'acné: rôle des hormones sexuelles dans sa physiopathologie et son traitement. Entretiens Bichat-Médecine, Expansion, Paris, p 695

Mauvais-Jarvis P, Kuttenn F (1976) Hirsutisme idiopathique: rôle respectif de l'hypersecrétion des androgénes et de leur métabolisme dans la peau. In: Scholler R (ed) Endocrinologie de l'ovaire. Sepe, Paris, p 449

Mauvais-Jarvis P, Bercovici JP, Gauthier F (1969) In vivo studies on testosterone metabolism by skin of normal males and patients with the syndrome of testicular feminization. J Clin Endocrinol Metab 29:417–421

Mauvais-Jarvis P, Bercovici JP, Crepy O, Gauthier F (1970a) Studies on testosterone metabolism in subjects with testicular feminization syndrome. J Clin Invest 49:31–40

Mauvais-Jarvis P, Guillemant S, Corvol P, Floch HH, Bardou L (1970b) Metabolism of radioactive 5α-androstane-3β, 17β-diol. Steroids 16:173–181

Mauvais-Jarvis P, Kuttenn F, Bercovici JP (1971) Tumeurs masculinisantes de l'ovaire. In: Decourt J, Dreyfus G (eds) Actual Endocrinol. Expansion, Paris, p 59

Mauvais-Jarvis P, Charransol G, Bobas-Masson F (1973) Simultaneous determination of urinary androstanediol and testosterone as an evaluation of human androgenicity. J Clin Endocrinol Metab 38:142–147

Mauvais-Jarvis P, Kuttenn F, Baudot N (1974) Inhibition of testosterone conversion to dihydrotestosterone in men treated percutaneously by progesterone. J Clin Endocrinol Metab 38:142–147

Mauvais-Jarvis P, Kuttenn F, Gauthier-Wright F (1976) Testosterone 5α-reduction in human skin as an index of androgenicity. In: James VHT, Serio M, Giusti G (eds) The endocrine function of the human ovary. Academic Press, New York, p 481

Mauvais-Jarvis P, Kuttenn F (1976b) Hirsutisme idiopathique: rôle respectif de l'hypersecrétion des androgénes et de leur métabolisme dans la peau. In: Scholler R (ed): Endocrinologie de l'ovaire. Sepe, Paris, p 449

Mauvais-Jarivs P, Kuttenn F, Lecomte P, Mandelbaum J (1977) Implication du systéme hypothalamo-hypophysaire dans le syndrome des ovaires polykystiques. In: Scholler R (ed) Exploration de l'unité hypothalamo-hypophysaire. Sepe, Paris, p 467

Mauvais-Jarvis P, Lecomte P, Kuttenn F, Mowszowicz I, Mandelbaum J, Gauthier-Wright F (1978) Etude hormonale compléte de 12 cas d'ovaires polykystiques type I. Ann Endocrinol (Paris) 39:191–199

Mauvais-Jarvis P, Kuttenn F, Mowszowicz I (1979) Androgen production and skin metabolism in idiopathic hirsutism. Recent results in peptide hormone and androgenic steroid research (Laszlo FA ed). Akademiai Klado, Budapest, p 223

McDonald P, Chapdelaine A, Gonzales O, Gurpide E, Van de Wiele RL, Lieberman S (1965) Studies on the secretion and interconversion of the androgens. III Results obtained after the injection of several radioactive C_{19} steroids singly or as mixtures. J Clin Endocrinol Metab 25:1557–1568

Meikle AW, Stringham JD, Wilson DE, Dolman LI (1979) Plasma 5α-reduced androgens in men and hirsute women: role of adrenals and gonads. J Clin Endocrinol Metab 48:969–975

Menon M, Tananis CE, Hicks LL, Hawkins EF, McLoughlin MC, Walsh PC (1978) Characterization of the binding of a potent synthetic androgen, methyltrienolone, to human tissues. J Clin Invest 61:150–162

Mercier-Bodard C, Baulieu EE (1968) Affinity of the testosterone-binding plasma protein for estradiol. C R Acad Sci[o] (Paris) 267:804–807

Mercier-Bodard C, Alfsen A, Baulieu EE (1965) A testosterone binding globulin. Excerpta Med Int Congr Ser 101:212–220

Mercier-Bodard C, Marchut M, Perrot M, Picard MT, Baulieu EE, Robel P (1976) Influence of purified plasma proteins on testosterone uptake and metabolism by normal and hyperplastic human prostate in "constant flow organ culture". J Clin Endocrinol Metab 43:374–386

Mercier-Bodard C, Renoir JM, Baulieu EE (1979) Further characterization and immunological studies of human sex-steroid binding plasma protein. J Steroid Biochem 11:253–259

Meyer III WJ, Migeon BR, Migeon CJ (1975) Locus on human X chromosome for dihydrotestosterone receptor and androgen insensitivity. Proc Natl Acad Sci USA 72:1469–1472

Michel G, Baulieu EE (1975) Androgen receptor in skeletal muscle. J Endocrinol 65:31–32

Moll GW, Rosenfield RL (1979) Testosterone binding and free plasma androgen concentrations under physiological conditions: characterization by flow dialysis technique. J Clin Endocrinol Metab 49:730–736

Moon YS, Tsang BK, Simpson C, Armstrong DT (1978) 17β-estradiol biosynthesis in cultured granulosa cells and theca cells of human ovarian follicles; stimulation by follicle stimulating hormone. J Clin Endocrinol Metab 47:263–267

Moore RJ, Wilson JD (1972) Localization of the reduced nicotinamide adenine dinucleotide phosphate: Δ_4–3-ketosteroid 5α-oxydoreductase in the nuclear membrane of the rat ventral prostate. J Biol Chem 247:958–967

Morfin RF, Di Stefano S, Bercovici JP, Floch HH (1978) Comparison of testosterone, 5α-dihydrotestosterone and 5α-androstane-3β, 17β-diol metabolisms in human normal and hyperplastic prostates. J steroid Biochem 9:245–252

Morris JM, Scully RE (1958) Endocrine pathology of the ovary. Mosby, St. Louis

Mowszowicz I, Bardin CW (1974) In vitro androgen metabolism in mouse kidney: high 3 keto-reductase (3α-hydroxysteroid dehydrogenase) activity relative to 5α-reductase. Steroids 23:793–807

Mowszowicz I, Bardin CW (1977) Effect of androgens and progestins on mouse kidney cells: an in vitro model distinct from that of intact kidney. Mol Cell Endocrinol 8:15–26

Mowszowicz I, Wright F (1979) A simple and reliable technique for separating the androgen receptor from TeBG in human tissues. Analytic Biochem 92:164–169

Mowszowicz I, Kahn D, Dray F (1970) Influence of testosterone binding to serum proteins on aromatization by enzymes of human placental microsomes. J Clin Endocrinol Metab 31:584–586

Mowszowicz I, Wright F, Bouchard P, Riahi M, Kuttenn F, Mauvais-Jarvis P (1979) Androgen receptor in human skin cytosol. 61st annual meeting of the American Endocrine Society. Anaheim, California: June, 13–15 Program and abstracts. Abstract no. 808

Mowszowicz I, Kirchhoffer MO, Kuttenn F, Mauvais-Jarvis P (1980) Testosterone 5α-reductase activity of skin fibroblasts: increase with serial subcultures. Mol Cell Endocrinol 17:41–50

Murphy BEP (1968) Binding of testosterone and estradiol in plasma. Canad J Biochem 46:299–302

Neumann F (1977) Pharmacology and potential use of cyproterone acetate. Horm Metab Res 9:1–13

Neumann F, Von Berswordt-Wallrabe R, Eiger W, Steinbeck H, Hahn JD, Kramer M (1970) Aspects of androgen-dependent event as studied by antiandrogens. Recent Prog Horm Res 26:337–405

New MI (1968) Congenital adrenal hyperplasia. Pediatr Clin North Am 15:395–407

New MI, Seaman MP (1970) Secretion rates of cortisol and aldosterone precursors in various forms of congenital adrenal hyperplasia. J Clin Endocrinol Metab 30:361–371

New MI, Lorenzen F, Pang S, Gunczler P, Dupont B, Levine LS (1979) "Acquired" adrenal hyperplasia with 21-hydroxylase deficiency is not the same genetic disorder as congenital adrenal hyperplasia. J Clin Endocrinol Metab 48:356–359

Newmark S, Dluhy RG, Williams GH, Pochi P, Rose LI (1977) Partial 11β- and 21-hydroxylase deficiencies in hirsute women. Am J Obstet Gynecol 127:594–598

Nikkari T, Valavaara M (1970) Effects of androgens on prolactin on the rate of production and composition of serum in hypophysectomized female rats. J Endocrinol 48:373–378

Nogeire C, Fukushima DK, Hellman L, Boyar RM (1977) Virilizing adrenal cortical carcinoma. Cancer 40:307–313

Northcutt RC, Island DP, Liddle GW (1969) An explanation for the target organ unresponsiveness to testosterone in the testicular feminization syndrome. J Clin Endocrinol Metab 29:422–425

Novak ER, Long JH (1965) Arrhenoblastoma of the ovary. Am J Obstet Gynecol 92:1082–1093

Novak ER, Woodruff JD (1974) Virilizing ovarian tumors. Gynecologia and obstetric pathology. (Novak ER, Woodruff JD Eds) Saunders, Philadelphia, p 469

O'Malley BW, Lipsett MB, Jackson MA (1967) Steroid content and synthesis in a virilizing luteoma. J Clin Endocrinol Metab 27:311–319

Panesar NS, Stitch SR (1976) Effects of cyproterone acetate on the biosynthesis of steroidal hormones. J Endocrinol 69:14–15

Parker CR, Servy E, McDonough PG, Mahesh VB (1974) In vivo endocrine studies in adrenal rest tumor of ovary. Obstet Gynecol 44:327–332

Pearlman WH, Crepy O (1967) Steroid protein interaction with particular reference to testosterone binding by human serum. J Biol Chem 242:182–189

Pearlman WH, Crepy O, Murphy M (1967) Testosterone-binding levels in the serum of women during the normal menstrual cycle, pregnancy and the post-partum period. J Clin Endocrinol Metab 27:1012–1018

Pham-Huu-Trung MT, Gourmelen M, Girard F (1973) The simultaneous assay of cortisol and 17α-OH progesterone in the plasma of patients with congenital adrenal hyperplasia. Acta Endocrinol (Copenh) 74:316–330

Pham-Huu-Trung MT, Gourmelen M, Raux-Eurin MC, Girard F (1978) Pituitary-adrenal-axis activity in treated congenital adrenal hyperplasia: static and dynamic studies. J Clin Endocrinol Metab 47:422–427

Photopulos GJ, McCartney WH, Walton LA, Staab EV (1979) Computerized tomography applied to gynecologic oncology. Am J Obstet Gynecol 135:381–383

Pinsky L, Kaufman M, Straisfeld C, Shanfield B (1974) Lack of difference in testosterone metabolism between cultured skin fibroblasts of human adult males and females. J Clin Endocrinol Metab 39:395–398

Pinsky L, Kaufman M, Straisfeld C, Zilahi B, Hall C (1978) 5α-reductase activity of genital and non genital skin fibroblasts from patients with 5α-reductase deficiency, androgen insensitivity or unknown forms of male pseudohermaphroditism. Am J Med Genet 1:407–416

Pochi PE, Strauss JS (1974) Endocrinologic control of the development and activity of the human sebaceous gland. J Invest Dermatol 62:191–201

Polansky S, de Papp EW, Ogden EB (1975) Virilization associated with bilateral luteomas of pregnancy. Obstet Gynecol 45:516–522

Prader A (1958) Die Häufigkeit des kongenitalen adrenogenitalen Syndroms. Helv Paediatr Acta 13:426–437

Prader A, Anders GJ, Habich H (1962) Zur Genetik des kongenitalen adrenogenitalen Syndroms. Helv Paediatr Acta 17:271–284

Proeschel MF, Courvalin JC, Donnadieu M, Binoux M, Girard F (1974) Preparation and evaluation of ACTH antibodies. Acta Endocrinol (Copenh) 75:461–477

Pujol A, Bayard F (1979) Androgen receptors in the rat epididymes and their hormonal control. J Reprod Fertil 56:217–222

Rager K, Huenges R, Gupta D, Bierich JR (1973) The treatment of precocious puberty with cyproterone acetate. Acta Endocrinol (Copenh) 74:399–408

Rebar R, Judd HL, Yen SSC (1976) Characterization of the inappropriate gonadotrophic secretion in polycystic ovary syndrome. J Clin Invest 57:1320–1329

Renoir JM, Fox LL, Baulieu EE, Mercier-Bodard C (1977) An antiserum specific for human sex steroid-binding plasma protein (SBP). FEBS Lett 75:83–88

Rice BF, Savard K (1966) Steroid hormone formation in the human ovary. Ovarian stromal compartment; formation of radioactive steroids from acetate $1-^{14}C$ and actions of gonadotropins. J Clin Endocrinol Metab 26:593–609

Riddick DH, Hammond CB (1975a) Long term steroid therapy in patients with adreno-genital syndrome. Obstet Gynecol 45:15–20

Riddick DH, Hammond CB (1975b) Adrenal virilism due to 21-hydroxylase deficiency in the post menarchial female. Obstet Gynecol 45:21–24

Rifka SM, Pita JC, Vigersky RA, Wilson YA, Loriaux DL (1978) Interaction of digitalis and spironolactone with human sex steroid receptors. J Clin Endocrinol Metab 46:338–344

Rivarola MA, Saez JM, Meyer WJ, Jenkins ME, Migeon CJ (1966) Metabolic clearance rate and blood production rate of testosterone and androst-4-ene-3, 17-dione under basal conditions, ACTH and HCG stimulation. Comparison with urinary production rate of testosterone. J Clin Endocrinol Metab 26:1208–1218

Rivarola MA, Singleton RT, Migeon CJ (1967 a) Splanchnic extraction and interconversion of testosterone and androstenedione in man. J Clin Invest 46:2095–2100

Rivarola MA, Saez JM, Jones HM, Jones GS, Migeon CJ (1967b) The secretion of androgens by the normal polycystic and neoplastic ovaries. Johns Hopkins Med J 121:82–90

Rivarola MA, Saez JM, Migeon CJ (1967c) Studies of androgens in patients with congenital adrenal hyperplasia. J Clin Endocrinol Metab 27:624–630

Robel P (1971) Steroid hormone metabolism in responsive tissues in vitro. Acta Endocrinol (Copenh) [Suppl] 153:239

Robel P, Lasnitzki I, Baulieu EE (1971) Hormone metabolism and action: testosterone and metabolites in prostate organ culture. Biochimie 53:81–96

Rose LI, Underwood RH, Williams GH (1973) Dihydrotestosterone formation in skin from different hair-bearing sites (Abstr.). Clin Res 21:482–483

Rosenfield RL (1971) Plasma testosterone binding globulin and indexes of the concentration of unbound androgens in normal and hirsute subjects. J Clin Endocrinol Metab 32:717–728

Rosenwaks Z, Lee PA, Jones GS, Migeon CJ, Wentz AC (1979) An attenuated form of congenital virilizing adrenal hyperplasia. J Clin Endocrinol Metab 49:335–339

Rosner W, Christy NP, Kelly WG (1969) Partial purification and preliminary characterization of estrogen binding globulins from human plasma. Biochemistry 8:3100–3108

Ryan KJ, Smith OW (1965) Biogenesis of steroid hormones in the human ovary. Recent Prog Hormone Res 21:367–409

Saez JM, Rivarola MA, Migeon CJ (1967) Studies of androgens in patients with adrenocortical tumors. J Clin Endocrinol Metab 27:615–623

Saitoh M, Uzuka M, Sakamoto M (1970) Human hair cycle. J Invest Dermatol 54:65–81

Sandberg EC, Jenkins RC, Trifon HR (1966) Biosynthetic studies of human ovarian arrhenoblastomous tissue in vitro. II. Formation of androgens from dehydroisoandrosterone sulfate. Steroids 8: 249–264

Sansone G, Reisner RM (1971) Differential rates of conversion of testosterone to dihydrotestosterone in acne and in normal human skin: a possible pathogenic factor in acne. J Invest Dermatol 56:366–372

Sarkar SD, Cohen EL, Beierwaltes WH, Ice RD, Cooper R, Gold EN (1977) New and superior adrenal imaging agent, ^{131}I-6β-iodomethyl-19-norcholesterol (NP-59): evaluations in humans. J Clin Endocrinol Metab 45:353–362

Sato T, Shinada T, Matsumoto S (1969) A clinical and metabolic study of masculinizing arrhenoblastoma. Am J Obstet Gynecol 104:1124–1130

Savard K, Gut M, Dorfman RI, Gabrilove JL, Soffer LJ (1961) Formation of androgens by human arrhenoblastoma tissue in vitro. J Clin Endocrinol Metab 21:165–174

Schaison G, Gilbert-Dreyfus (1974) Hyperplasie surrénale congenitale a révélation tardive; à propos de trois cas de déficit en 11β-hydroxylase. Ann Med Int (Paris) 125:163–168

Scully RE (1963) Androgenic lesions of the ovary. In: Graay HG, Smith DE (eds) The ovary. Williams & Wilkins, Baltimore, p 143

Seabold JE, Schteingart DE (1975) I-131- iodocholesterol imaging in adrenal neoplasm (Abstr.). J Nucl Med 16:566

Shanies DD, Hirschhorn K, New MI (1972) Metabolism of testosterone-^{14}C by cultured human cells. J Clin Invest 51:1459–1467

Shearman RP, Cox RI (1966) Enigmatic polycystic ovary. Obstet Gynecol Surv 21:1–12

Short RV, London DR (1961) Defective biosynthesis of ovarian steroids in the Stein-Leventhal syndrome. Br Med J 1:1724–1727

Shuster E, Leake FM (1968) Luteoma of pregnancy. Obstet Gynecol 32:637–642

Siiteri PK, Wilson JD (1974) Testosterone formation and metabolism during male sexual differentiation in the human embryo. J Clin Endocrinol Metab 38:113–124

Sitruk-Ware R, de Lignières B, Basdevant A, Mauvais-Jarvis P (1980) Absorption of percutaneous estradiol in post-menopausal women. Maturitas, Elsevier Holland, 2:207–211

Slaunwhite WR, Sandberg AA (1959) Transcortin: a corticosteroid binding protein of plasma. J Clin Invest 38:384–391

Snochowski M, Pousette A, Ekman P, Bression D, Anderson L, Högberg B, Gustafsson JA (1978) Characterization and measurements of the androgen receptor in human prostatic hyperplasia and prostatic carcinoma. J Clin Endocrinol Metab 45:920–930

Southren AL, Gordon GG, Tochimoto S (1968) Further studies of factors affecting the metabolic clearance rate of testosterone in man. J Clin Endocrinol Metab 28:1105–1112

Southren AL, Gordon GG, Tochimoto S, Krikun E, Krieger D, Jacobson M, Kuntzman R (1969 a) Effect of N-phenylbarbital (Phetarbital) on the metabolism of testosterone and cortisol in man. J Clin Endocrinol Metab 29:251–256

Southren AL, Gordon GG, Tochimoto S, Olivo J, Sherman DH, Pinzon G (1969 b) Testosterone and androstenedione metabolism in the polycystic ovary syndrome: studies on the percentage binding of testosterone in plasma. J Clin Endocrinol Metab 29:1356–1363

Steeno D, Heyns W, Vanbaelen H, Demoor P (1968) Testosterone binding in human plasma. Ann Endocrinol (Paris) [Suppl 29] 29: 141–148

Steg A, Benoit G, Limouzin-Lamotte A (1979) Percutaneous 17β-estradiol in the treatment of prostatic cancer. 9th Meeting int study group for steroid Horm 11 Rome 5–1 December. Program and Abstracts. Abstract no. 20, to be published by Pergamon Press in 1981

Stein IF Jr, Leventhal ML (1935) Amenorrhea associated with bilateral polycystic ovaries. Am J Obstet Gynecol 29:181–191

Stern AP, Brown BW, Haskell WL, Farqhar JW, Wehrle CL, Wood PD (1976) Cardiovascular risk and use of estrogens or oestrogenprogestagen combinations. Stanford three community study. J Am Med Ass 235:811–815

Sternberg WH, Barclay DL (1966) Luteoma of the pregnancy. Am J Obstet Gynecol 95:165–184

Sternberg WH, Dhurandar HN (1977) Functional ovarian tumors of stromal and sex cord origin. In: Scully RE, Robby SJ (eds) Human pathology. Saunders, Philadelphia, p 565

Stewart ME, Pochi PE, Strauss JS, Wotiz HH, Clark SJ (1977) In vitro metabolism of ^{3}H-testosterone by scalp and back skin: conversion of testosterone into 5α-androstane-3β, 17β-diol. J Endocrinol 72:385–390

Strauss JS, Pochi PE (1963) The human sebaceous gland: its regulation by steroidal hormones and its use as an end organ for assaying androgenicity in vivo. Recent Prog Horm Res 19:385–444

Strauss JS, Kligman AM, Pochi PE (1962) The effect of androgens and estrogens on human sebaceous glands. J Invest Dermatol 39:139–155

Strott CA, Yoshimi T, Lipsett MB (1969) Plasma progesterone and 17-hydroxyprogesterone in normal men and children with congenital adrenal hyperplasia. J Clin Invest 48:930–939

Sullivan JN, Strott CA (1973) Evidence for an androgen-independent mechanism regulating the levels of receptor in target tissue. J Biol Chem 248:3202–3208

Svensson J, Snochowski M (1979) Androgen receptor levels in preputial skin from boys with hypospadias. J Clin Endocrinol Metab 49:340–345

Symington T (1963) The pathology of the adrenal hyperactivity. Br J Urol 35:329–341

Tait JF, Horton R (1966) The in vivo estimation of blood production and interconversion rates of androstenedione and testosterone and the calculation of their secretion rates. In: Pincus G, Nakao T, Tait JF (eds) Steroid dynamics. Academic Press, New York, p 393

Takayasu S, Adachi K (1972) The conversion of testosterone to 17β-hydroxy-5α-androstan-3-one (dihydrotestosterone) by human hair follicles. J Clin Endocrinol Metab 34:1098–1101

Takayasu S, Adachi K (1975) The intranuclear binding of 17β-hydroxy-5α-androstan-3-one and testosterone by hamster sebaceous gland. Endocrinology 96:525–529

Thomas JP, Oake RJ (1974) Androgen metabolism in the skin of hirsute women. J Clin Endocrinol Metab 38:19–22

Thomas PZ, Dorfman RI (1964) Metabolism in vitro of androst-4-ene-3, 17-dione-4-^{14}C by rabbit skeletal muscle strips. J Biol Chem 239:762–765

Tomkins GM (1956) A mammalian 3α-hydroxysteroid dehydrogenase. J Biol Chem 218:437–447

Touitou Y, Bogdan A, Legrand JC, Desgrez P (1977) Metabolisme de l'OP'DDD (Mitotane) chez l'homme et chez l'animal. Ann Endocrinol (Paris) 38:13–25

Touitou Y, Bogdan A, Luton JP (1978) Changes in corticosteroid synthesis of the human adrenal cortex in vitro induced by treatment with OP'DDD for Cushing's syndrome: evidence for the sites of action of the drug. J Steroid Biochem 9:1217–1224

Tulchinsky D, Chopra IJ (1974) Estrogen-Androgen imbalance in patients with hirsutism and amenorrhea. J Clin Endocrinol Metab 39:164–169

Valette A, Carasco G, Verine A, Varesi L, Boyer J (1978) Differential effects of oestradiol and ethinyloestradiol on lipid metabolism in the female rat. J Endocrinol 79:405–406

Van Baelen H, Heyns W, de Moor P (1969) Microheterogeneity of the testosterone binding globulin of human pregnancy serum demonstrated by isoelectric focusing. Ann Endocrinol (Paris) 30: 199–203

Verhoeven GFM, Wilson JD (1979) The syndromes of primary hormone resistance. Metabolism 28:253–289

Vermeulen A, Ando S (1979) Metabolic clearance rate and interconversion of androgens and the influence of the free androgen fraction. J Clin Endocrinol Metab 48:320–325

Vermeulen A, Verdonck L (1968) Studies on the binding of testosterone to human plasma. Steroids 11:609–635

Vermeulen A, Verdonck L (1978) Sex hormone concentrations in post-menopausal women. Relation to obesity, fat mass, age and years post-menopause. Clin Endocrinol (Oxf) 9:59–66

Vermeulen A, Verdonck L (1976) Plasma androgens levels during the menstrual cycle. Am J Obstet Gynecol 125:491–494

Vermeulen A, Verdonck L, Van der Straeten M, Orie N (1969) Capacity of the testosterone-binding-globulin in human plasma and influence of specific binding of testosterone on its metabolic clearance rate. J Clin Endocrinol Metab 29:1470–1480

Vermeulen A, Stoica T, Verdonck L (1971) The apparent free testosterone concentration, and index of androgenicity. J Clin Endocrinol Metab 33:759–767

Vigersky RA, Loriaux DL, Howards SS, Hodgen GB, Lipsett MB, Chrambach A (1976) Androgen binding proteins of testis, epididymis and plasma in man and monkey. J Clin Invest 58:1061–1068

Voigt W, Hsia SL (1973) Further studies on testosterone 5α-reductase of human skin. J Biol Chem 248:4280–4285

Voigt W, Fernandez EP, Hsia SL (1970) Transformation of testosterone into 17β-hydroxy-5α-androstan-3-one by microsomal preparations of human skin. J Biol Chem 245:5594–5599

Weiland AJ, Bookstein JJ, Cleary RE, Judd HL (1978) Preoperative localization of virilizing tumors by selective venous sampling. Am J Obstet Gynecol 131:797–802

Wentz AC, White RI Jr, Migeon CJ, Hsu TH, Barnes HV, Jones GS (1976) Differential ovarian and adrenal vein catheterization. Am J Obstet Gynecol 125:1000–1007

Werk EE, Sholiton LJ, Kalejs L (1973) Testosterone secreting adrenal adenoma under gonadotropin control. N Engl J Med 289:767–770

West CD, Atcheson JB, Stanfield JB, Rallison ML, Chavre VJ, Tyler FH (1979) Multiple or single 21-hydroxylases in congenital adrenal hyperplasia. J Steroid Biochem 11:1413–1419

Wiechert R (1967) Synthesen anti-androgenen steroide. In: Raspe G (ed) Advances in the biosciences. Pergamon, New York, p 54

Wieland RC, Vorys N, Folk RL, Hamwi GJ (1967) Urinary testosterone fraction. Am J Obstet Gynecol 99:489–496

Wiest WG, Zander J, Holmstrom EG (1959) Metabolism of progesterone 4-C^{14} by an arrhenoblastoma. J Clin Endocrinol Metab 19:297–305

Wilkins L, Gardner LI, Crigler JF Jr, Silverman SH, Migeon CJ (1952) The control of hypertension with cortisone with a discussion of variations in the type of congenital adrenal hyperplasia and report of a case with probable defect of carbohydrate regulating hormones. J Clin Endocrinol Metab 12:1015–1030

Wilson EA, Erickson GF, Zarutski GF, Zarutski P, Finn AE, Tulchinsky D, Ryan KJ (1979) Endocrine studies of normal and polycystic ovarian tissues in vitro. Am J Obstet Gynecol 134:56–63

Wilson JD (1975) Dihydrotestosterone formation in cultured human fibroblasts. Comparison of cells from normal subjects and patients with familial incomplete male pseudo-hermaphroditism type 2. J Biol Chem 250:3498–3504

Wilson JD, Walker JD (1969) The conversion of testosterone to 5α-androstan-17β-ol-3-one (dihydrotestosterone) by skin slices of man. J Clin Invest 48:371–379

Witschi E (1963) Embryology of the ovary In: Grady HG, Smith DE (eds) The ovary. Williams & Wilkins, Baltimore, p 1

Wotiz HH, Mescon E, Doppel H, Lemon HM (1956) The in vitro metabolism of testosterone by human skin. J Invest Dermatol 26:113–120

Wright F, Giacomini M (1980) Reduction of dihydrotestosterone to androstanediols by human female skin in vitro. J Steroid Biochem 13:639–643

Wright F, Kirchhoffer MO, Mauvais-Jarvis P (1976) Antagonist action of dihydroprogesterone on the formation of the specific dihydrotestosterone cytoplasmic receptor complex in rat ventral prostate. 5th Int. Congress Endocrinol, Hamburg. July 18–24. Abstracts of short communications and poster presentations p 149. Abstract no 362.

Wright F, Mowszowicz I, Mauvais-Jarvis P (1978) Urinary 5α-androstane-3α, 17β-diol radioimmunoassay: a new clinical evaluation. J Clin Endocrinol Metab 47:850–854

Wright F, Kirchhoffer MO, Mauvais-Jarvis P (1979) Antagonist action of dihydroprogesterone on the formation of the specific dihydrotestosterone-cytoplasmic complex in rat ventral prostate. J Steroid Biochem 10:419–422

Wright F, Kirchhoffer MO, Giacomini M (1980) Antiandrogenic activity of progesterone in human skin. In: Mauvais-Jarvis P, Vickers CFH, Wepierre J (eds) Percutaneous absorption of steroids. Academic Press, London, pp 123–137

Yamaji T, Dierschite DJ, Hotchkiss AN, Bhattacharva AN, Surve AH, Knobil E (1971) Estrogen induction of LH release in the Rhesus monkey. Endocrinology 89:1034–1041

Yen SSC, Vela P, Rankin J (1970a) Inappropriate secretion of follicle stimulating hormone and luteinizing hormone in polycystic ovarian disease. J Clin Endocrinol Metab 30:435–442

Yen SSC, Vela P, Ryan KJ (1970b) Effect of clomiphene citrate in polycystic ovary syndrome: relationship between gonadotropin and corpus luteum function. J Clin Endocrinol Metab 31:7–13

Yen SSC, Chaney C, Judd HL (1976) Functional aberrations of the hypothalamic pituitary system in polycystic ovary syndrome: a consideration of the pathogenesis. In: James VHT, Serio M, Giusti G (eds) The endocrine function of the human ovary. Academic Press, New York, p 373

Zachman M, Prader A (1980) Clinical and biochemical variability in congenital adrenal hyperplasia (CAH) due to 11β-hydroxylase deficiency. 6th Int Congr Endocrinology, Melbourne. 10–16 February. Program and Abstracts p 583 Abstract 148.

Zieger G, Lux B, Kubatsch B (1976) The effect of cyproterone acetate on the adrenal of the male hamster. Acta Endocrinol (Copenh) 82:127–133

Zourlas PA, Jones HW Jr (1969) Stein-Leventhal syndrome and masculinizing ovarian tumors. Obstet Gynecol 34:861–866

Subject Index

Adrenal
  congenital adrenal hyperplasia 43
  hirsutism of adrenal origin 43
  virilizing tumours 54
Adrenocorticotrophic hormone (ACTH)
  stimulative test 34, 37
Anagen 3
Androgen
  biosynthetic pathways 5
  control of production 9
  interconversions 5
  mode of action 18–30
  origin of circulating androgens in women 7–8
  production rates 5
  transport of blood 11
Androstanediols
  biological evaluation 40–41, 78
  origin and circulation in blood 9
  physiological importance 26
Androstenedione
  dihydrotestosterone formation from androstenedione 26, 77–78
  origin and circulation in blood 9
Antiandrogens
  cyproterone acetate 86–90
  oestrogen 83–85
  progesterone 85–86
Assays
  in blood 35–40
  in urine 33–35, 40
Arrhenoblastoma 67–69

Binding
  intracellular binding of androgen to receptor 27–30
  other plasma binding globulins 12
  testosterone binding globulin (TeBG) 11–13
Biological assessment of hirsutism 33–42
Biosynthesis of androgens 5

Catheterization (see vein)
Clinical assessment of hirsutism 31–33
Clomiphene citrate, test in polycystic ovarian syndrome 61–62
Congenital adrenal hyperplasia
  due to 21-hydroxylase defect 43–53

  due to 11β-hydroxylase defect 53–54
Cortisol treatment of congenital adrenal hyperplasia 52–53
Corticosteroids, treatment of hirsutism with 91
Cyproterone acetate, treatment of idiopathic hirsutism 86–90

Dehydroisoandrosterone (free and sulfate)
dihydrotestosterone formation from dehydroisoandrosterone 26
in virilizing adrenal tumors 56–57
  origin and circulation 6–9
  plasma assays 39
Delayed onset congenital adrenal hyperplasia 47–50
Dexamethasone suppressive tests 34, 37
Dihydrotestosterone
  intracellular metabolism 26–27
  intracellular retention 27–31
  origin and circulation in blood 9
  plasma assays 39
  5α-reduction of testosterone to dihydrotestosterone 19–26
Dynamic tests 34–39

Enzyme defect (see congenital adrenal hyperplasia)
  Oestradiol test in polycystic ovarian syndrome 62
Oestrogen
  oestrogen-androgen balance in woman 13
  production in polycystic ovarian syndrome 65
  treatment 83–85

Ferriman and Gallway method 31
Fibroblasts, cultured skin 24–26, 28–29

Genetic of congenital adrenal hyperplasia 50–51
Genital skin, androgen metabolism 22
Gonadotropins
  dynamic tests 34, 37
  in polycystic ovarian syndrome 60–61
Granulosa cell tumours 68

Hair growth 2–3
Hepatic metabolism 15
Hilus cell tumours 67
Hirsutism
 clinical assessment 31–33
 hormonal investigation 33–42
 idiopathic 74–82
 of adrenal origin 43–59
 of ovarian origin 60–73
 treatment 82–91
HLA group system in congenital adrenal hyperplasia 51
Hormonal investigation of hirsutism 33–42
Hydroxylase
 21-hydroxylase defect 43–53
 11β-hydroxylase defect 53–54
Hyperplasia (see congenital adrenal hyperplasia)
Hyperthecosis, ovarian 72

Idiopathic hirsutism
 basis of 74
 clinical and biological characteristics 76–81
 hypersensitivity versus androgen overproduction 75–76
 treatment 81, 83–90
Interconversion of androgens 5
Intracellular
 metabolism of androgens 19–26
 retention of dihydrotestosterone 27–31
Investigation (see hormonal)

Ketosteroid, urinary 17-ketosteroids 57
LH-RH test in polycystic ovarian syndrome 61
Lipid cell tumours 67
Luteoma 67

Mechanism of action of androgens in human skin
 androgen receptor 29
 dihydrotestosterone formation 26
 intracellular retention of dihydrotestosterone 26–31
 5α-reductase of testosterone 19–26
Metabolic clearance rate of androgen 16–17
Metabolism
 of androgen in human skin 19–26
 of androgen in the liver 15
Mitotane (see OP'DDD)

OP'DDD, treatment of adrenal cancer 58–59
Origin of circulating androgens
 in hirsute women 47–49, 56–57, 77–80
 in normal women 5–10

Ovarian (Hirsutism of ovarian origin)
 hyperthecosis 72
 ovarian tumours 66–72
 polycystic ovarian syndrome 60–66
 treatment 72

Percutaneous oestrogen treatment 86–90
Pilosebaceous gland, control 2–3
Plasma androgen assay (see androgen and assays)
Polycystic ovarian syndrome
 clinical 60–61
 hormonal 61–64
 pathophysiology 64–66
Progesterone, treatment of hirsutism 85–86
Pubic skin, androgen metabolism 20

Receptor, of androgen (physicochemical characteristics) 28–30
Receptivity, of skin to androgens 18–30, 74–76
Reductase
 3-keto reductase in skin 26–27
 5α-reductase activity in human skin 19–26

Skin androgen control of pilosebaceous gland 2–3
 metabolism of androgens 19–26
 receptors 27–31
Steroids (see androgen, oestrogen, cortisol)
Suppressive tests
 with dexamethasone 34, 37
 with oestrogen 34, 37

Testosterone
 origin and circulation in blood 8, 13
 metabolism in liver 15
 metabolism in skin 19–22
 mode of action at cellular level 29
 assays 35–36
Testosterone binding globulin (TeBG) 11–13
Tests
 clomiphene test in polycystic ovary 61–62
 dynamic tests 34–39
 LH-RH test in polycystic ovary 61
 of adrenal function 34
 of ovarian function 34
Treatment of hirsutism
 idiopathic 81
 methods (see also antiandrogen) 83–91
 of adrenal origin 52–53, 58–59,
 of ovarian origin 72

Vellus 2
Vein catheterization 38, 58, 70

Other Volumes in This Series:

Volume 18: I. J. Chopra
Triiodothyronines in Health and Disease
With a Contribution by V. Cody
1981. 72 figures, 18 tables. IX, 145 pages
ISBN 3-540-10400-3

Volume 17: J. Chayen
The Cytochemical Bioassay of Polypeptide Hormones
1980. 72 figures, 7 tables. XIV, 208 pages
ISBN 3-540-10040-7

Volume 16: J. E. A. McIntosh, R. P. McIntosh
Mathematical Modelling and Computers in Endocrinology
1980. 73 figures, 56 tables. XII, 337 pages
ISBN 3-540-09693-0

Volume 15: A. T. Cowie, I. A. Forsyth, I. C. Hart
Hormonal Control of Lactation
1980. 64 figures, 7 tables. XIV, 275 pages
ISBN 3-540-09680-9

Volume 14: J. H. Clark, E. J. Peck, Jr.
Female Sex Steroids
Receptors and Function
1979. 116 figures, 18 tables. XII, 245 pages
ISBN 3-540-09375-3

Volume 13: H. F. DeLuca
Vitamin D – Metabolism and Function
1979. 14 figures. VIII, 80 pages
ISBN 3-540-09182-3

Volume 12
Glucocorticoid Hormone Action
Editors: J. D. Baxter, G. G. Rousseau
1979. 176 figures, 58 tables. XIX, 638 pages
ISBN 3-540-08973-X

Volume 11: S. Ohno
Major Sex-Determining Genes
1979. 34 figures, 6 tables. XIII, 140 pages
ISBN 3-540-08965-9

Volume 10: W. I. P. Mainwaring
The Mechanism of Action of Androgens
1977. 12 figures, 17 tables. XI, 178 pages
ISBN 3-540-07941-6

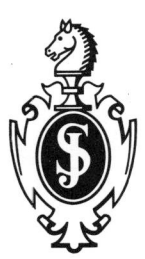

Springer-Verlag
Berlin
Heidelberg
New York

Volume 9: R. E. Mancini
Immunologic Aspects of Testicular Functions
1976. 36 figures, 8 tables. IX, 114 pages
ISBN 3-540-07496-1

Volume 8: E. Gurpide
Tracer Methods in Hormone Research
1975. 35 figures. XI, 188 pages
ISBN 3-540-07039-7

Volume 7: E. W. Horton
Prostaglandins
1972. 97 figures. XI, 197 pages
ISBN 3-540-05571-1

Volume 6: K. Federlin
Immunopathology of Insulin
Clinical and Experimental Studies
1971. 53 figures. XIII, 185 pages
ISBN 3-540-05408-1

Volume 5: J. Müller
Regulation of Aldosterone Biosynthesis
1971. 19 figures. VII, 137 pages
ISBN 3-540-05213-5

Volume 4: U. Westphal
Steroid-Protein Interactions
1971. 144 figures. XIII, 567 pages
ISBN 3-540-05312-3

Volume 3: F. G. Sulman
Hypothalamic Control of Lactation
In collaboration with numerous experts.
1970. 58 figures. XII, 235 pages
ISBN 3-540-04973-8

Volume 2: K. B. Eik-Nes, E. C. Horning
Gas Phase Chromatography of Steroids
1968. 85 figures. XV, 382 pages
ISBN 3-540-04277-6

Volume 1: S. Ohno
Sex Chromosomes and Sex-linked Genes
1967. 33 figures. X, 192 pages
ISBN 3-540-03934-1

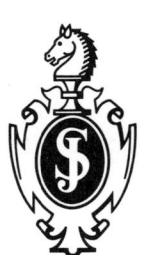

Springer-Verlag
Berlin
Heidelberg
New York

DATE DUE